1 11.99

YOGA FOR M

THE WEISER CONCISE GUIDE SERIES

YOGA

FOR

MAGICK

NANCY WASSERMAN

EDITED AND INTRODUCED BY
JAMES WASSERMAN

WEISERBOOKS
San Francisco, CA / Newburyport, MA

First published in 2007 by
Red Wheel/Weiser, LLC
With offices at:
500 Third Street, Suite 230
San Francisco, CA 94107
www.redwheelweiser.com

ISBN-10: 1-57863-378-8
ISBN-13: 978-1-57863-378-4
Library of Congress Cataloging-in-Publication Data
available upon request

Cover design by Maija Tollefson
Book design by Studio 31
www.studio31.com

Typeset in Adobe Sabon
Cover photograph © Ordo Templi Orientis

Printed in Canada
TCP
10 9 8 7 6 5 4 3 2 1

To

Jim, Rachel, Satra

Emma, Amir, Illia, Bill T.,

Bill B., and Genevieve:

my fellow passengers on the bus.

CONTENTS

ACKNOWLEDGMENTS

I HAVE BEEN A STUDENT OF THE OCCULT for many years. This book is the result of the experiments and experiences—both sublime and disastrous—that I have encountered along the way. However, I could not have produced this work without the help and encouragement I received from my colleagues and family.

My husband, James Wasserman, is an exacting and careful editor. He managed to wade patiently through revision after revision as I brought my message into crisper focus. I very much appreciate both his assistance and his patience as he helped me juggle responsibilities on many different levels while I worked on this book.

My daughter Rachel cheerfully shared her time and allowed me the necessary space to complete this project. However, she never allowed her mom to get too serious and knew exactly when to pull her out into the sunshine to play.

Emma Gonzalez graciously agreed to pose for the photographs presented in this book. The energy she brings into her practices are evident even in these still photos.

Thanks to Merigene Riggins for her gentleness and encouragement as well as her intelligent perspective.

Thank you, Leroy Lauer, for your keen eye for detail.

Bill Thom, Gwen Cummings, Genevieve Mikolajczak, and Stella Grey helped refine this work and make it suitable for a wider audience.

My brother Kent Finne lent his always unique perspective to this book.

I appreciate the efforts of Donald and Yvonne Weiser, Mike Conlon, and Zoe Mantarakakis, as well as the enthusiasm of Brenda Knight.

Thanks to J. Daniel Gunther for his kind words and support: they are precious to me.

Special thanks are due to Lynn Scriven who kindly lent her careful and practiced eye to this text. Her suggestions and observations are invaluable and her comments have strengthened this book considerably.

Any omissions or oversights that may occur in this book are my own responsibility.

INTRODUCTION
by

JAMES WASSERMAN

Yoga for Magick is written for the student of Western esotericism—the Magician or Wiccan who might be least likely to buy a book on Yoga. The truism that "necessity is the mother of invention" should help give it context. Think of this as a rule book for becoming healthy, wealthy, and wise, especially wise. If you practice the techniques you find here, in six months you won't recognize yourself, especially on a spiritual level.

It is the author's contention, and I agree, that aspiring adepts of the Western Mystery Traditions are often less likely to be concerned with concentration, meditation, and the overall health and flexibility of the physical body than they should be. This book provides a practical means of correcting that problem. You will be led step-by-step through the age-old wisdom of Yoga and meditation in a well-reasoned series of discussions and instructions—as devoid as possible of the cultural anomalies so common to most other Yoga books. This is truly intended to be Yoga for Magicians and, we might add, Witches, Pagans, Qabalists, and others who follow the Western Paths of Attainment.

Here are some thoughts on why I believe it is necessary to build a stronger foundation for most of the traditions that make up modern Western occultism. I have enjoyed considerable interactions with Yogis, Sufis, Buddhists, and Wiccans, as well as adherents of the Magical Path. In 1976, some eight-and-a-half years after committing my life to the Holy Spirit, I joined a fraternal magical order of which I am still a member. Destiny, perhaps, put me in wider contact with more disparate groups of seekers on the spiritual path than is common.

While undisciplined generalization is one of the cardinal sins of thought, processing information into recognizable patterns is one of the cardinal virtues of rationality. Thus it is with a mixture of trepidation and confidence that I make the following statement. Based on my own observation, a startling number of practitioners of Western systems such as Magick and Wicca tend to be less concerned with physical health than students of other spiritual disciplines.

One is more likely to encounter overweight people, chronic users of tobacco, those unduly indulging in intoxicants, and students less concerned with diet, exercise, muscle tone, and flexibility than one should expect. This is somewhat incomprehensible. I have found the most challenging demands made on my physical vehicle by the energies associated with Magick. I have also been forced by my magical practices to continuously refine (sometimes dramatically) my relationship to the needs of my body. Advancing age now plays no small part in bringing to awareness the critical necessity of working against entropy in order to remain spiritually flourishing.

The physical body is the living temple of the Holy Spirit. A person who can't sit in one position with comfort and quiet, who can't breathe with evenness and regularity, who can't temporarily still the mind of its many warring thoughts, and who can't channel powerful energies through the body because of ill health—will be hard-pressed to spiritually advance.

Nancy Wasserman has included an accurate and valuable summary of the history of Yoga in the West, focusing especially on the occult revival of the late nineteenth- and early twentieth-century magical orders. In my opinion, the primary nexus point of the spread of these Teachings in modern culture was the phenomena of the 1960s and more specifically the use of LSD by many of my generation. Raised on *Lassie* and *The Lone Ranger*, we were catapulted into the fourth dimension by a liquid spot on a piece of paper or cube of sugar. With no preparation, a number of people experienced advanced—if thoroughly chaotic—states of mind, to which many experienced adepts, who had done the work unaided by the miracle of modern chemistry, felt we were not entitled. Introduction to such psychic realms had been reserved for millennia to patient chelas of demanding gurus who had painstakingly mapped out pathways of consciousness and rules of behavior for those who sought after such mysteries.

There were immediate consequences. The stoned-out hippies of Woodstock were replaced by pool-cue-wielding Hell's Angels at Altamont. Baba Ram Dass was preaching love and meditating in India while Charlie Manson's "Family" was committing horrors I am loathe to describe. As Brian Jones, Jimi Hendrix, Janis Joplin, and Jim Morrison died in rapid succession and at roughly the same age, we knew something was wrong. The explosive deaths of three members of the Weathermen revealed a communist bomb factory in a wealthy Greenwich Village townhouse. The sociopath Eldridge Cleaver imprisoned Timothy Leary, himself widely accused of being a government agent. Then John Lennon was shot; Abbie Hoffman committed suicide; and now Ozzy Osbourne, Sean Penn, and Courtney Love serve as contemporary poster people for the admonition, "This is your brain on drugs." The '60s are here officially declared not only dead, but buried.

I met an adept named Adano Ley in 1972. He told me he spent many hours each night on the Inner Planes working with others at his level to clear up the chaos that had been created in the Universal Mind by psychedelic drugs. He may have been crazy, or we may owe him a good deal of gratitude for his efforts. The point is that a sea change occurred in the

West. Aleister Crowley predicted it in a letter to Grady McMurtry, later Caliph Hymenaeus Alpha of Ordo Templi Orientis. Crowley wrote in 1945 that some twenty years hence he expected a radical transformation in consciousness to occur. Crowley's particular influence in creating it (by, among other things, introducing Aldous Huxley to mescaline) was significant.

The purpose of these reflections is to give some context for my initial observation that many of those who follow a Western Magical Path may be less inclined to accept the rigors of physical culture than they should be. The specifics of our Tradition are less mature than those of the imported Traditions to which so many other seekers have been attracted. In other words, when a Maharishi or Swami teaches in the West, his students get Indian rules and guidance that have remained in place for three thousand years or more. What to eat, how to exercise, when to sleep, what clothes to wear.

We, on the other hand, have been told "Do what thou wilt shall be the whole of the Law" (or some variant such as "An harm ye none, do what you will"). That ain't much in the way of guidance folks—relatively speaking of course! Couple this with the breakdown of the Western family that has raged out of control since ... the 60s ... and you begin to get a picture of the need for some basic advice on the how-tos of successfully living life and pursuing Spiritual Wisdom. And this is what, I am delighted to say, runs through this book on nearly every page.

Here you will learn to enlist your body as an ally in the quest for spiritual growth. There are instructions in the proper positions for meditation. Easy to understand breathing exercises are given that will form the perfect platform for more advanced practices. Different mantras are suggested and their use is carefully explained. Step-by-step directions in progressively more advanced meditation techniques will be found here that take the practitioner on a well-planned path of sustainable conscious development. The theoretical underpinnings of why these techniques work are also explained. In addition, Nancy offers a particularly helpful discussion of diet and the basics of healthy living from both her own scientific research and personal lifestyle. Her discussion of the moral and behavioral aspects required for an aspirant to progress along the spiritual path is invaluable as a springboard for personal contemplation of one's true role in the world.

Finally she includes two detailed practices designed to help the reader implement these teachings in a particularly energizing manner.

The first is a magical exercise that deals with raising occult power through the body and improving health on both a physical and spiritual level. It is perhaps the key Western ritual for strengthening the aura. And the reader will discover that its origins are firmly rooted in Yoga.

The second involves a series of daily invocations combined with Yoga postures. The exercises are illustrated with photographs, and are designed to simultaneously stretch and strengthen the body, while psychically attuning the student to the magical rhythms of Nature.

If you follow what is offered in these pages with some diligence, this book can help you become the adept you dream of becoming. I truly hope it will.

OVERVIEW

Magick is a Pyramid, built layer by layer.
The work of the Body of Light, with the technique
of Yoga, is the foundation of the whole.

ALEISTER CROWLEY[1]

THE WORD *Yoga* connotes many different images: from wizened holy men meditating in caves to perfectly proportioned health-club denizens arranged in neat rows eager to try out the latest craze. *Yoga* means "union" and is linked etymologically with the English word "yoke."

Yoga is a multidimensional discipline designed to help the individual achieve a state of health, serenity, focus and, ultimately, union with the Divine. The practice of Yoga in the East extends far back to the beginnings of civilization. Many schools of yogic philosophy have developed over the centuries, but essentially five points remain consistent in all disciplines of Yoga today. According to Swami Sivananda, one of the foremost proponents of Yoga in the West, these five principals are: proper exercise, proper breathing, proper relaxation, proper diet, and positive thinking and meditation.

Yoga is a close cousin of Magick and both disciplines have the same purpose: to increase wisdom, to explore the Self, to attain higher levels of consciousness, and, ultimately, to attain that spiritual state known in the West as the Knowledge and Conversation of the Holy Guardian Angel. Both Yoga and Magick allow their adherents to open themselves as conduits for divine expression.

Obviously, the first question is this: If both paths lead to the same point, why is it important for a Western Magician to practice Yoga? The answer lies in Yoga's holistic approach to attainment. Yoga affects all levels of a person's being: starting with the skin and muscles and penetrating to the deeper realms of the psyche, endowing him with the tools necessary to accomplish his goals. The physical health, discipline, and concentration skills gained through the practice of Yoga are essential to the practice of Magick and the development of the Body of Light.

The form of Yoga discussed in this book is known as *Ashtanga,* or the "Yoga of Eight Limbs." These eight limbs are *Yama, Niyama, Asana, Pranayama, Pratyhara, Dharana, Dhyana,* and *Samadhi.*

Yama and Niyama, knowledge of the moral principles of behavior, along with simple contemplation, lend the necessary serenity and introspection to begin the practices. They are time-honored ways of calming the mind and making the student aware of the results of actions both on himself and others.

Asanas, the body positions of Hatha Yoga, give control over the physical body. Asana and Hatha Yoga lend the physical strength, flexibility, and general good health necessary to function optimally in the outside world. Being in good physical health makes available the stamina required to work efficiently on magical levels. The asanas also prevent a myriad of health problems: from obesity to endocrine issues, to bone and joint disorders, and many others.

Pranayama strengthens the nervous system, allowing it to adapt to stressors in an efficient manner. Besides boosting the immune system, Pranayama is calming and cleansing to the aura. Steady practice of Pranayama sharpens the magical intent.

Pratyhara, Dharana, and Dhyana deal with the ability to empty the mind of outside thought and concentrate on a single object or purpose. This is the essential condition to magical success.

Pratyhara teaches the ability to resolutely withdraw from the senses and shut down all impressions from the outside. It demands control over action, speech, and thought. It will rid the mind of random impulses and drifting mental processes.

Dharana involves concentration techniques essential to the practical Magician, which train the mind to focus on a single point.

Dhyana goes a step further. It may be considered a result of Dharana. One becomes conscious of the union of subject and object, the true underlying identity of ourselves with the object of our concentration.

Samadhi is the state one enters when all outside perceptions and consciousness are dropped. Samadhi may be achieved by any person who succeeds at Yoga. May all attain!

I have also included information on the Chakras, or energy centers, which are central to the practitioner's spiritual health. Chakras are an important component of both Western and Eastern psychic maps. The Middle Pillar exercise in the appendix celebrates the marriage of the yogic Chakras with the Qabalistic spheres.

Mantra Yoga is also discussed because of its integral relationship with Pranayama and its usefulness during ritual. Repetition of sacred chants uplifts the soul, allows the mind to focus on a single stream of thought, and may be used to regulate the breath.

My primary spiritual experiences stem from my work in the Western magical system, and specifically from my study of the works of Aleister Crowley and his teaching of Thelema, the exploration of the True Will. I am also a member of Ordo Templi Orientis, the largest Thelemic organization in the world. While the text of this book reflects my interest in Crowley's thought, the techniques are equally valid and useful for anyone on the Western path regardless of whether you identify yourself as a Witch, Neopagan, Wiccan, Golden Dawn adherent, Chaos Magician, or any other variation of the mystical path. Understanding the basic elements of Yoga: developing the necessary skills to sit quietly and comfortably, breathe evenly, and still the mind for a period of time are necessary to the successful spiritual practice of any aspirant.

This book emphasizes the five points of Yoga mentioned earlier: proper exercise, proper breathing, proper relaxation, proper diet, positive thinking and meditation. These essential pursuits are often overlooked by modern esotericists. We are always in a rush to get where we are going. Yoga teaches us to slow down, concentrate, and pay attention to the silence.

NANCY WASSERMAN
New York City
2006

PART ONE

YOGA IN THEORY

CHAPTER ONE

THE ORIGINS OF YOGA

Every form in this world is taken out of
surrounding atoms and goes back to these atoms.
Law is uniform; nothing is more certain than that.
If this is the law of nature, it also applies to
the mind. The mind will dissolve and
go back to its origin.

VIVEKANANDA[2]

THE PRACTICE OF YOGA is as ancient as Hindu culture.
Although it is an ever-evolving practice, Yoga's origin is the
Indus Valley civilization of South Asia, which flourished
around 2500 B.C. Spanning what is now Pakistan and western India, the Indus Valley was home to the largest of the
four ancient urban civilizations (in addition to Egypt,
Mesopotamia, and China). It was an area rich with culture
and sophisticated religious practice.

The first written records of the doctrines of Yoga are in
the Vedic literature of the Aryans (ca. 3000–1200 B.C.).
These philosophies were first referenced in the classical text,
the Upanisads. The Upanisads (literally meaning "sit down
near") are also known as the Vedantas, or the last of the
Vedas, the ancient hymns of knowledge. They are considered
the core treatises of orthodox Hindu philosophy and wisdom
teachings.

The Bhagavad-Gita was written in approximately 600
B.C. Part of the extraordinary Mahabharata, the Bhagavad-
Gita is a dialogue between Lord Krishna and the war-
rior prince Arjuna expounding the philosophies of Yoga.
Gautauma Buddha was living and teaching at about the same

time. Yogic practices were assimilated into Buddhism and the wisdom teachings spread throughout Asia.

Some four hundred to six hundred years later, at the dawn of the common era (somewhere between 200 B.C. and 200 A.D.), *The Yoga Sutras of Patanjali* was written. *Yoga Sutras* is considered to be the classic Yoga text. Patanjali described in detail the eight parts of Ashtanga Yoga on which most modern Yoga practices are based. These eight "limbs" are:

1. Yama: Guidelines for interactions with others.
2. Niyama: Guidelines for managing and purifying oneself.
3. Asana: A practice of using physical postures to gain self-discipline and physical health.
4. Pranayama: Breathing techniques focused on control and awareness of the connection between breath, mind, and the emotions.
5. Pratyhara: Techniques aimed at withdrawal or detachment from the senses.
6. Dharana: A concentration technique in which the attention is focused on a single point.
7. Dhyana: Contemplation; A keen awareness without focus on any thought or object; the single point of Dharana has been brought down to zero and one glimpses the truth behind the veil of matter.
8. Samadhi: Transcendence of self and union with the Divine.

Around the time of the European Middle Ages, the classic *Hatha Yoga Pradipka* was written. Hatha Yoga was originally designed to prepare the mind for meditation. The ancient sages taught that only through the physical discipline of Hatha could the mind and nervous system be prepared for the challenging task of mental stillness.

In Europe there is little evidence of the knowledge of yogic practices until the Theosophical Society started publishing some of the works of Patanjali in the 1800s. In 1897, Swami Vivekananda published his classic *Raja-Yoga*. Also in 1895, Karl Kellner established the Ordo Templi Orientis, which provides a synthesis of Eastern and Western wisdom teaching. However, we suspect that Yoga practices were taught long before on a one-to-one basis, and that methods to improve single-pointed concentration have always been circulated among occultists.

At the turn of the twentieth century, several factors lent themselves to the wider dissemination of Yoga in the West. The Golden Dawn was attracting some notable members, including the exceptionally talented Alan Bennett. Bennett was well versed in both Western and Eastern techniques and was especially drawn to yogic practices. He met Aleister Crowley when Crowley joined the Golden Dawn in 1898; the two men became friends and Bennett took Crowley under his wing, teaching him basic meditation and magic techniques. Bennett suffered from chronic asthma and, with Crowley's help, relocated to Ceylon for his health.

In Sri Lanka, Bennett was able to take advantage of formal Yoga training. Upon his arrival, he was hired as a tutor to the son of the solicitor general of Ceylon, P. Ramathan. Ramathan was profoundly knowledgeable in Eastern religious practices. Bennett studied Yoga with him and learned a great deal about its theory and practice. In 1901, Crowley joined Bennett for a magical retreat in Kandy where Bennett instructed him in yogic philosophy and technique. Eventually, Bennett was ordained a Buddhist priest and later became one of the founders of the Buddhist movement in the West. Crowley published two notable works on Yoga and they remain some of the most concise, practical instruction available to the Western esoteric student. Part 1 of Crowley's *Magick: Liber ABA, Book Four* (referred to later in this text as *Magick: Book Four*) was first published in 1912 and his *Eight Lectures on Yoga* was published in 1939.

Today, there are many different schools of Yoga. Hatha Yoga is widely accepted and is taught all over the world. Besides finding instruction in dedicated Yoga schools and ashrams, one can find Hatha Yoga taught in hospitals, community centers, gyms, and churches. The health benefits of meditation are also recognized; one can find instruction almost anywhere. Offshoots of classical meditation, such as visualization, are gaining wide popularity as millions of people with widely divergent interests discover the benefits of regular practice of these time-honored physical and mental techniques.

Where does this leave the modern occultist? We have never been better positioned to take advantage of Yoga. Even though the most valuable experiences will be those initiated and practiced in the privacy of our temples, beginners have access to a wide variety of excellent resources for instruction. More experienced Magicians can find new ways of deepening their practice.

CHAPTER TWO

YOGA AS A PHYSICAL DISCIPLINE

... a well-trained body helps a great deal to train the mind, which is the main purpose of all Yoga, in order to attain complete freedom and immortality, which is the aim of all religions of the world.

SWAMI VISHNUDEVANANDA[3]

WHAT? This is a book for *Magicians*! Why should Magicians be concerned about cultivating a physical discipline? Many people on the magical path believe the work of magical ritual is not necessarily carried out on a physical plane but on the inner planes. Why should they worry about health? If Magicians need to spend time cultivating the "body of light," why bother with the body of flesh?

In fact, many people involved in spiritual pursuits tend to neglect their physical condition. Yet there are numerous distinguished voices that echo a different sentiment. Take for example Dion Fortune, who wrote this in the 1930s:

The occultist aims at making his physical body a vehicle that shall impede him as little as possible in his psychic activities. That is to say, it must be as refined as possible, using the word in the metallurgist's sense, not the social sense. Secondly, it must be of a strength and toughness to be able to endure the exceptional forces he requires it to transmit. The adept therefore is not an etherealized person, like the conventional saint in a stained glass window. A trained occultist is, by virtue of his training, capable of great physical endurance and exceedingly tenacious of life, as is witnessed by the extraordinary happenings in connection with the murder of the infamous Rasputin, who resisted cyanide of potassium and bullets through the heart and brain, and had finally to be literally hacked to pieces before life was extinct.[4]

While most Western adepts would agree that a person does not need to go to the lengths of some of the Yogis in India, in the discipline of Magick it is very important to possess general good health and a strong and flexible body.

In today's world, it is quite easy to ignore the body. Hungry? Stick something in the microwave or hit the "drive-thru" or fast-food restaurant on the way home from work and pick up some dinner. Little creative thought or energy goes into preparing it, and people tend to just as carelessly choke it down. Such food, which usually has an abundance of sugar, salt, and preservatives, adds unhealthy weight and diminishes vitality: a lethal combination in the practice of Magick. A generation of American children remain enthroned upon their couches watching television while munching potato chips. Let us instead be about the work of establishing temples and honing magical skills.

Students of the occult, like all students, are inclined to do a lot of reading and thinking, intellectually exploring the universe. While this may be an admirable trait, it is very important not to neglect other aspects of life. Taking the time to cook a good meal, clean the house, or weed the garden is as important to magical development as sketching that Enochian tablet. Sometimes the subconscious mind needs a break to process the information one is so painstakingly gathering.

DIET AND THE SPIRITUAL PATH

Concerning food, there are no hard and fast rules about diet among Western occultists. Unlike traditional yogic proscriptions, it is not considered taboo to eat red meat, drink alcohol, or even to imbibe other mind-altering substances. Indeed, if you are devoting a magical operation to a particular deity, you may actually feel it necessary to consume certain things foreign to your upbringing or your basic nature. In my experiences though, I have found the Gods are kind and generally allow compromise: Let your intuition guide you in your choices. In all matters concerning diet, let it be known that moderation is the key. While tobacco is considered the primary perfume of Horus, a smoker with lung cancer would be of little benefit to Him. Addiction, weakness, and disease form no part of His vigorous nature. Nor would one be serving Jupiter by feasting to the point of obesity, heart disease, or diabetes mellitus. Any excessive action one may feel required to explore or endure for the purpose of invocation should be performed on a short-term basis only. Remember the words *delicacy*, *subtlety*, and *discrimination*. In contrast, Yoga has clear dietary guidelines. And Magicians should be conscious of the dietary choices they are making. These guidelines from the yogic path may be used as a springboard to thinking about one's personal choices. It is as important to discover what is the best fuel for the body as it is to discover the specifics of one's practical moral code.

The body has often been referred to as "the temple of the soul." Food is one of the body's sacraments. As such, regardless of whether the student is a strict vegetarian, an omnivore, or anything in between, it is of absolute importance to give the body good food. Observe how the body reacts to different types of foods. Decide what your approach to alcohol should be. Be brutally honest. Reevaluate your needs from time to time. For example, although I had been a vegetarian for several years, I found it necessary to add fish back into my diet while I was expecting my daughter. The demands of pregnancy were such that I required the type of energy produced by consuming fish.

The typical yogic diet is lacto-vegetarian. It consists of whole grains, legumes, vegetables, fruits, seeds, nuts, and dairy products. It bans eggs or flesh of any kind. This diet is very important to Yogis for both moral and health reasons. While externally it is very wholesome and simple, it takes into account the subtle effects foods have on both Prana (energy) and the mind. Dietary choices are intertwined with spiritual choices. Many Yogis believe that the mind is formed from the minute, ethereal essence of food. So optimally, any food the Yogi consumes is as pure as possible.

Yoga divides food into one of the three basic classifications, or *gunas*. The three gunas represent the different vibratory essences of the energies of creation. They are *sattvic*, pure; *rajasic*, active; and *tamasic*, dark. The gunas correspond to the Western alchemical principles of Mercury, Sulphur, and Salt. The gunas characterize the intrinsic nature of all things existing on earth including people. Yogis believe that a person's mental makeup will be influenced by the types of food he eats.

Sattvic foods are the choice of most Yoga practitioners. They are considered to enhance prana and to increase strength, cheerfulness, and joy. Sattvic foods maximize vitality, energy, vigor, health and happiness. They are both delicious and nutritious. They are believed to grant calmness, supply maximum energy, and boost stamina. They are conducive to the practice of meditation and magical studies. The traditional categorizations of the foods are listed below; again, let your intuition guide you in dietary choices.

- Legumes, seeds, and nuts are essential to the yogic diet. They contain high amounts of protein needed to build muscle and strength.
- Whole grains such as steel cut oats, corn, millet, quinoa, unpolished rice, and barley are considered a mainstay. These types of grain are beneficial for the entire digestive system, from the jaws to the elimination processes. Grains supply carbohydrates that lend energy to the body as well as providing amino acids that help form the building blocks of protein.
- Fresh vegetables contain necessary minerals, vitamins, and fiber. Yogis consume a variety of vegetables, including leafy greens, root vegetables, and vegetables with seeds (like squash or cucumbers). All products should be as fresh as possible and cooked as lightly as possible.
- Fruits are considered one of the most important parts of the yogic diet. All types of fruit are included: whether fresh, dried, or juiced. They have a high vitamin and mineral content and are considered vitalizing. They are also thought to be blood purifiers, which is the reason it is common for Yoga adherents to fast for periods of time, drinking only fruit juices. It is acceptable to dilute juices with pure spring or natural, bubbling mineral water. I would especially recommend this modification for those sensitive to sugar or wishing to drop excess weight.
- Herbs are used both as seasoning and as tisanes.
- All sweeteners should be as natural as possible: honey, molasses, maple syrup, and apple juice concentrate are preferred. Do not eliminate sweets, but enjoy them in moderation. Jaggery, which is

raw unprocessed sugar obtained directly from sugar cane, is a traditional sweetener in India. It is becoming more commonly available today in both the United States and Europe.

• Traditionally, dairy products such as milk, butter, cheese, and yogurt were considered an important part of the sattvic diet. Today, however, due to modern farming practices, many feel more comfortable using alternatives such as soy or rice products. Another drawback to dairy products is that they are believed to increase the production of mucus in the body, which could have an impact on breathing exercises.

Rajasic foods are salty, bitter, overly hot, pungent, burning, sour and/or dry. They tend to excite passions and produce a rather ineffective, overly active disposition. The yogic diet avoids them because they are overly stimulating and can cause both physical and mental stress. Rajasic foods incite lust, anger, greed, violence, and other vices thought to hinder the practitioner in his studies. On a mundane level, rajasic foods can cause insomnia and irritation of the GI tract. It has been my observation that many occultists (including myself!) are attracted to rajasic comestibles. Foods classified as rajasic include:

• Onions, garlic, radishes, coffee, tea, tobacco, or any type of stimulant
• Salty foods
• Excessively spicy food
• "Convenience" food laden with chemicals and preservatives
• Soft drinks
• Mustard
• Pungent spices (such as asafetida)

- White sugar (considered overly processed)
- Sattvic food eaten too quickly ("on the go")

Tamasic foods are tasteless, putrid, rotten, and stale. This type of food makes a person listless, sluggish, and indolent. Tamasic food brings on feelings of anger and depression; the mind becomes inappropriately dark and filled with the residue of disappointments. Abandoning this type of food can bring dramatic changes in the psyche. Tamasic foods include:

- Meats, fish, eggs, alcohol, and all other intoxicants
- Stale, rotten, or decomposed foods
- Overripe or underripe fruit
- Fermented food
- Deep-fried food, overly barbecued food ("charred"), or food that has been reheated many times
- Mushrooms and other fungi
- Vinegar
- Sattvic food taken in excessive quantity

Regardless of the type of diet you choose, make any changes or adjustments slowly and aim toward simplicity. Remember, the goal is to make the body so supple, strong, healthy, and comfortable that one is able to *ignore* it through the course of magical practices. Sudden changes and complicated regimes tend to make one more *conscious* of the body, the exact opposite of the goal. Try to make the diet as well-balanced as possible. Do not eat too much or too little. One needs as much energy and vigor as possible for magical work. Improper eating habits lead to physical and mental characteristics not compatible with the Great Work.

Respect your food. Pause before eating to say a simple prayer of gratitude or a few words of acknowledgment and intent. Even if one is amongst a crowd, a silent recitation of prayer or intent uplifts a simple meal to a higher level. Remember Aleister Crowley's words in *Magick: Book Four*, "Every intentional act is a magical act."

PHYSICAL DISCIPLINE AND THE SPIRITUAL PATH

The other half of the physical culture equation is physical exercise. It is very important for occultists to be strong in body, intellect, and psyche because of the powerful nature of the energies involved in performing ritual Magick. Efforts devoted to improving health will in turn afford more time and energy for occult work.

Although any form of athleticism will be beneficial, I personally feel that Hatha Yoga is an excellent choice for occultists as it provides benefits systemically. Its approach is a holistic one that can reduce chronic musculoskeletal pain, decrease weight, and tone muscle. Yoga helps to regulate the endocrine system and is especially beneficial for people who suffer with diabetes or thyroid disorders. It can relieve mild depression and anxiety. And, of course, Yoga reduces stress. Research suggests it may even be helpful to those with obsessive-compulsive disorders.

Certain types of breathing exercises (Pranayama) benefit the physical body. Besides the obvious advantages of clearing nasal passages and eliminating excess mucus, particular breathing exercises help to strengthen the abdominal wall. Any Pranayama exercise that involves forceful exhalation—such as *Kapalabhati* (described later in the chapter on Pranayama)—provides a workout for the deeply placed *transversus abdominus* muscle. This is the muscle you use when coughing, sneezing, or forcibly exhaling. Since it doesn't move the spine, the transversus abdominus does not engage when doing exercises, like "crunches."

The benefits of flexibility, focus, and stress reduction are very attractive and useful tools for the practicing Magician. In addition, the asanas practiced in Hatha Yoga are thought to help purify the mind's psychic realms. They help to open up the *nadis*, the body's subtle energy channels, that allow the *Kundalini*, the life force and psychic energy, to flow freely. Hatha Yoga is also a perfect way to begin and/or end a meditation session. It is definitely an optimal way to "warm up" prior to any type of ritual work, energizing the muscles, heart, lungs, and psyche simultaneously.

How exactly does one start a Hatha Yoga practice? The first thing to do, and sometimes the hardest, is to find a suitable teacher. There are many different types of Hatha Yoga available. It is wise to start with a little research into the different schools and classes available in your area, ranging from the purposeful approach of Iyengar style Yoga to the intense physicality of Bikram Yoga. Look for word-of-mouth referrals. There are usually classes offered at gyms or through city recreation departments. There may be an ashram or dedicated Yoga center in a location nearby. Try as many different styles as possible. Having an actual certified, trained teacher available is very important.

Remember that the whole point of Yoga is knowing and accepting who you are at the moment. Yoga is not about competition. Do not strain while doing Hatha Yoga; steady practice will bring steady improvement.

You'll also need a thin foam mat from either a Yoga supply store or camping goods store. This will protect the spine when bending and performing the various postures. The best type of mat to purchase is known as a "sticky" mat. These mats provide traction to the floor as well as the feet, making them safer to use. You can find sticky mats for sale almost anywhere Yoga supplies are sold as well as in some department stores.

In Appendix Two, "Solar Workings" we give instruction on an exercise known as the Salutations to the Sun (*Soorya Namaskar*). The solar sphere is associated with health and vitality, as well as devotion to the Great Work. While the poses in the series are relatively simple, the Sun Salutation completely stretches and strengthens all parts of the body, including arms, legs, and the entire spine. It is a great way to regain and improve natural flexibility and encourage relaxation, focus, and centering.

The Sun Salutation becomes especially interesting when combined with Liber Resh vel Helios, a magical solar adoration also included in the "Solar Workings" appendix. One might start the Sun Salutation exercise by saying Liber Resh aloud, and then visualizing the appropriate images throughout the various postures. Combining the Yoga Sun Salutation with Liber Resh will strengthen resolve toward the Great Work.

In addition to Hatha Yoga, I've had profound experiences from my involvement with dance. Dance is an effective way to connect with the Divine and a very handy skill for dramatic ritual. Dance gives suppleness, poise, and balance, which are very desirable traits to cultivate for magical practices. Aleister Crowley writes the following in *Magick: Book Four* regarding the nature of circumambulations:

> A particular tread seems appropriate to it. This tread should be light and stealthy, almost furtive, and yet very purposeful. It is the pace of the tiger who stalks the deer....

> Another important movement is the spiral, of which there are two principal forms.... In the spiral the tread is lithe and tripping almost approximating to a dance, while performing it the Magician will usually

turn on his own axis, whether in the same direction as the spiral, or in the opposite direction....

There is also the dance proper; it has many different forms, each God having his special dance. One of the easiest and most effective dances is the ordinary waltz-step combined with the three signs of L.V.X. It is much easier to attain ecstasy in this way than is generally supposed.[5]

The motor coordination and agility provided by both dance and Yoga can be of great benefit to the occultist. Awareness of the physical body as a projection of the True Will is a key to wisdom. Magicians make maps of the universe and the physical plane is part of that universe. Intimate understanding of both the skills and limitations of the exterior physical self is as important as knowledge of the interior, astral, or akashic states. One doesn't necessarily have to become a triathlete or marathon runner, but it is important to maintain your physical health.

If Yoga or dance don't suit your personality, try the martial arts. Tai Chi is especially beneficial. I have also spoken with people who enjoy running. They state that the release of endorphins experienced during a morning jog inspire them in their ritual endeavors. Regardless of your choice, regular practice of a physical discipline will improve your ability to perform spiritual work.

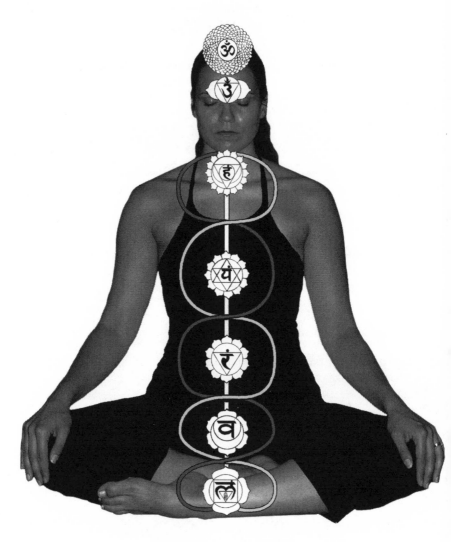

Chakras in descending order:
At the top of the head is *Sahasrara;*
at the eyebrows is *Ajna;* at the throat is *Vishuddha;*
at the heart is *Anahata;* at the solar plexus is *Manipura;*
at the genitals is *Svadishthana;* and at the base is *Muladhara.*
The *Sushumna* nadi is the vertical channel;
the *Ida* nadi is shown in white; the *Pingala* nadi is shown in gray.

CHAPTER THREE

CHAKRAS: THE WHEELS OF LIGHT

*The occultist does not regard the brain as
the vehicle of mind, but rather as the organ of
motor coordination and sensation: a very
different matter. For him, the vehicles
of mind are the seven chakras.*

DION FORTUNE[6]

Chakras are best described as energy centers. They are the
psychic hubs through which the spiritual energy of Kundalini
is moved and charged as it rises through the body. When one
becomes conscious of the chakras through visualization,
Pranayama, and Mantra Yoga, they become centers of transformation and catalysts for spiritual evolution.

The five lower chakras: the *Muladhara, Svadhisthana,
Manipura, Anahata,* and *Vishuddha:* are associated with the
five *tattwas* or elements: earth, water, fire, air, and ether
(akasha). The *Ajna* chakra contains a combination of the
purified forms of all the tattwas, while the *Sahasrara* chakra
is considered to function beyond the realm of the tattwas.

Each of the elements has corresponding strengths and
weaknesses within the physical body. According to the his-
torical texts, the changes produced by the rhythmic currents
of the chakras' psychic energy produce physical changes
within the body. Because these elements ebb and flow following the natural rhythmic patterns of the body, great attention and emphasis is given to the chakras both in yogic
practice and Auryvedic medicine.[7] These changes in chemical
makeup are very similar to what Western science explains
today as the action of the endocrine glands.

For the Magician, exploration and knowledge of the chakras provide a valuable map to the personal psychic realm. It is possible to actually sense and "see" the Kundalini energy passing through the chakras and circulating within the body. Becoming more conscious of the chakras is also an invaluable tool for centering and strengthening the Body of Light. In Appendix One, we have provided an excellent Qabalistic ritual/meditation called the Middle Pillar, for magical work with the chakras.

The flow of psychic energy between the chakras and within the body is conducted through the subtle channels, or nadis. The three most important nadis are called *Ida*, *Pingala*, and *Sushumna*. One can become more aware of them through meditation. They can also function as conduits of magical power during ritual. The Sushumna is considered the primary nadi. It originates in the Muladhara chakra (the base chakra), along with Ida and Pingala, and moves straight upward through the spinal column. Sushumna then splits: the anterior branch terminates in the Ajna chakra at the pineal gland, and the posterior branch travels behind the skull, ending in the area of the anterior fontanel.

Sushumna has been described as multicolored and "shining like jewels." Sushumna carries the major force of magical energy through the chakras. Ida and Pingala also rise toward the Ajna chakra, but their movement is serpentine. They move around the chakras instead of passing directly through them like Sushumna.

Ida is located on the left side of Sushumna. Usually described as pale and luminous, it carries lunar currents and is considered feminine in nature. Energies moving through Ida are constructive, life-sustaining, and maternal. Ida is connected with the prana flowing in and out of the left nostril. This energy is thought to be particularly purifying and creative. Concepts to keep in mind when working with Ida include purity, magnetism, femininity, the visual sense, emotion, and creative energy.

Pingala is located on the right side of the Sushumna. Its primary characteristics are solar and masculine. It's color is described as red. Pingala is connected with the prana flowing in and out of the right nostril. The energies carried through the Pingala nadi are considered destructive. Pingala purifies by fire. Key words to remember when thinking of Pingala are electricity, masculinity, the verbal faculty, rationality, vigor, and dynamic energy.

After exiting and separating at the Muladhara chakra, the three nadis conjoin once more at the Ajna chakra. They create a knotlike form, which the Yogis call *Mukta Triveni*. *Mukta* means "liberated." This is significant because if one is able to raise the Kundalini into and through Mukta Triveni, one is said to move beyond the confines of time. Past, present, and future open to the adept and he or she is liberated from the bondage of reincarnation.

Take a careful look at the descriptions of the chakras. While one or two will likely resonate more profoundly than the others, it is important to explore each center systematically. You will discover more than you ever thought possible about your personality and potential.

The Muladhara Chakra

The Muladhara chakra is located in the sacral (base) area of the spine near the perineum. This chakra is predominated by a *yantra*[8] in the shape of a large four-sided figure, whose color is traditionally listed as orpiment, a sulfuric orange-yellow. This yantra has one large red petal on each side. In the center of the yantra is a red triangle representing triple energy. Inside the triangle is the sacred life force, the shining

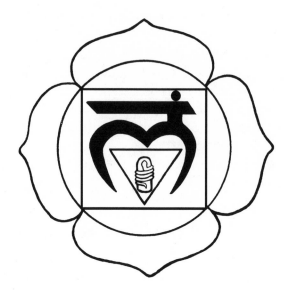

Muladhara Chakra

serpent Kundalini, coiled around the *Svayambhu Lingam.*[9]
This energy is aroused by the intensity of the Yogi's focus.
The upward-pointing lingam and coiled serpent suggest an
ascending movement, the natural flow of energy toward the
Sahasrara chakra.

The secret symbol or *bija* mantra[10] associated with the
Muladhara chakra is the Sanskrit letter *Lang.* This mantra is
pronounced by squaring the lips and tongue, and placing the
tongue against the palate. You should feel a vibration on the
palate and the sinus cavities. Repetition of the bija is said to
remove material insecurities and to bring inner awareness.
This mantra also prevents any downward flow of Kundalini.
When chanting any of the bija mantras, it is useful to place
the center of your focus on the physical location of the corresponding chakra.

Meditation and mantra centered on the Muladhara
are associated with issues about self-identity, security, pos-

sessions, fears, and inhibitions. Because the Muladhara is associated with the element of Earth, or *Prithvi,* basic needs such as food, shelter, warmth, and a safe environment are of concern.

Working magically with the energies of the Muladhara chakra unlocks the door to progressively higher states and an awareness of the massive potential of the Kundalini energy stored within. Concentration on this chakra will also help the Magician formulate, stabilize, and accept his approach to the sensual realms.

The Svadhisthana Chakra

The Svadhisthana chakra is visualized as a six-petaled lotus with a shining crescent in the center. It is located near the genitalia, above the Muladhara center in the pelvic region. Its color is a pearlescent white, traditionally described as being

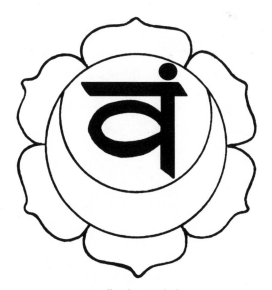

Svadhisthana Chakra

"like a conch shell." This chakra has six petals of an orange-red color. Its seed mantra is *Vam,* and its tattwa is *Apas,* or Water. The emotional nature is the primary quality of this chakra.

The shell-like color may be a reference to the conch shell held by Vishnu, the presiding deity of Svadhisthana. Vishnu represents the power of preservation. It is fitting that his seat is in the center of sexual energy. Mantra and meditation on this chakra are associated with sexuality, ripeness, smoothness, joy, trust, the unconscious mind, the astral plane, and imagination. There is also a sense of divine grace, as well as activation of creative and sustaining energy within the Yogi. While meditation on Svadhisthana bestows an abundance of creativity and desires, success in this center also brings a level of control over the passions: One should be able to make appropriate choices and separate fantasy from reality.

The Manipura Chakra

The Manipura chakra is located in the solar plexus or umbilical region. The yantra in the center of the chakra is a red downward pointing triangle, symbolic of *Agni,* the tattwa associated with Manipura, the descending fire of inspiration. Think of lightening strikes from the sky.[11] The ten dark blue petals surrounding this chakra represent the energizing nerve centers of the body, and are described as the ten pranas (vital breaths) of Shiva. The bija color is described as a golden yellow, which is why people sometimes think that the primary color of this chakra is yellow. The bija mantra is *Rang.*

Meditation on the Manipura center brings a decreased sense of egoism and the power to shape, create, and change one's life. Because working in this sphere brings a sense of open-mindedness, a person's capacity for enjoyment, jovial-

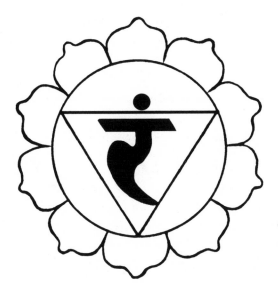

Manipura Chakra

ity, and passion are increased. The capacity for bliss and courage are also enhanced by attention to this chakra. A person becomes better able to articulate his or her thoughts and can bring the visualizations formulated in Svadhisthana into practical application. The power to direct and regulate psychic energy is enhanced in Manipura as well.

When an occult practitioner, whether a Witch, Magician, or Yogi, decides to "center" himself, he or she usually focuses on the alignment of the chakras with both the earth and heavens. During that process, it is highly effective to sense the Manipura center as the center point between the chakras, while visualizing oneself as the center point between the heavens and earth.[12]

Meditation on Manipura helps develop understanding of human physiology, especially the endocrine glands. It is said that concentration on this chakra will improve the function of the gastrointestinal system. When the Manipura is well-developed, great amounts of vitality may be drawn from food.

The Anahata Chakra

The Anahata chakra is located in the region of the heart, at the thoracic cavity, in front of the spinal column and behind the breastbone. Traditionally, it is said to be clear or color-less, although some authorities describe it to be a smoky gray or smoky green color. The bija mantra of Anahata is *Yang*. The yantra of Anahata is visualized as a hexagram composed of an upward and a downward pointing triangle, which in this system represents *prana vayu*, vital life breath, or air. This air, so important in the function of the heart and lungs, moves prana throughout the body. In Anahata, the energies are balanced and flowing in all directions. The message of

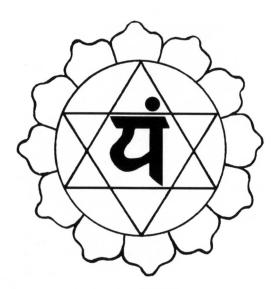

Anahata Chakra

the fourth chakra is harmony on the internal and external planes.

One should strive to have intimate knowledge and awareness of the heartbeat during Anahata meditation and rituals, paying attention to its rates and rhythms. Work in this center helps to create self-generating, self-emanating energy. Creativity can be enhanced in Anahata as well: art created on this plane is attuned with the rhythm of the heart, the rhythm of the universe. True comprehension of the concept of *Bhakti* Yoga, the Yoga of devotion (described in depth by Aleister Crowley in Liber Astarté vel Berylli) rests here. Meditation on this chakra also brings a sense of balance to the physical, rational, emotional, and sensual aspects of the personality. It also helps the adept to discover, cultivate, and apply inner strength.

The Vishuddha Chakra

The Vishuddha chakra is known as the voice of the heart. All genuine forms of communication, both verbal and nonverbal, originate here. Vishuddha is located at the base of the throat and is visualized as a silvery, pale purple crescent within a shining white circle, enclosed by sixteen lotus petals. Both the crescent and the shimmering circle encompassing it are reflective of the lunar nature of Vishuddha: cloudless psychic energy, clairvoyance, and the ability to decipher unspoken, extrasensory messages. The secret symbol or bija mantra of this chakra is *Ham.*

Vishuddha is considered to be cooling and operates only on the highest levels. Vishuddha means "pure" and is the center of divine love. All true mystics and inspired artists are said to operate on this plane. The spoken word originates here as do great art and poetry.

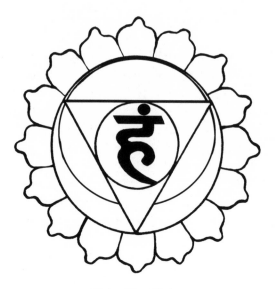

Vishuddha Chakra

The element associated with this chakra is *Akasha*, also known as ether or "antimatter." It is the element most closely tied with the astral plane. Vishuddha is related to memory, witticism, intuition, and improvisation: all of which manifest from Akasha.

Meditation on Vishuddha is the beginning of the path of knowledge that leads to divine awareness. The earthly elements dissolve as one enters the realm of cosmic consciousness or *chit*. At this level the adept is granted calmness, purity, serenity, a beautiful voice, and a command of speech. It is said one will be able to understand the mantras, obtain the ability to compose poetry, decipher the message of dreams, and interpret holy scriptures. Because it deals with purity, concentration on this center may grant the capacity to be a careful and honest spiritual teacher.

The Ajna Chakra

The Ajna chakra is located in the space between the eyebrows, at the pineal gland. It is described as being transparent camphor blue to luminescent white in color. During meditation, it appears in the form of a two-petaled lotus. The bija mantra associated with Ajna is *Aum*, the experience of divine energy. The element corresponding to Ajna is *mahat tattwa*, the purified essence of all the tattwas. It is from this tattwa that all the other elements emerge.

Meditation on Ajna is said to eliminate sins and impurities and to give visions of the past, present, and future. Ajna brings the gift of truth. The person who has opened himself to truth sees divinity reflected in every living thing. Those who become centered within the Ajna chakra rise above the common elements.

The Ajna center is also believed to be the place where thoughts originate, and these thoughts are the key to magical endeavors. Both subconscious and conscious thoughts influence the direction of one's magical workings. Focus on activating the Ajna center can benefit a practitioner by bestowing higher thought patterns and the ability to see things objectively, thus creating a fuller understanding of the motives behind actions.

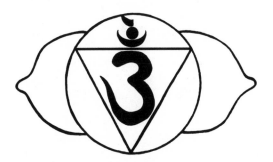

Ajna Chakra

By working with the energies of the Ajna chakra, the Yogi or Magician can rise above the concepts of time and the basic desires that cause a person to act in mundane matters. One may experience an objective realization of truth. Uncovering the mysteries of Ajna allows the practitioner to move higher still. For beyond the Ajna is Sahasrara.

Sahasrara Chakra

This is the creation of the world, that the pain of division is as nothing, and the joy of dissolution all.

THE BOOK OF THE LAW

The Sahasrara chakra is located at and slightly above the crown of the head, encompassing the cranial plexus. While some texts state that this chakra is formless, it is elsewhere described as resembling a full moon. Above the sphere is a vast canopy of a thousand lotus petals in every color imaginable. On each of the petals is inscribed one of the fifty Sanskrit letters. In the Sanskrit system, each letter represents a nadi, or energy channel. These letters are repeated endlessly on the many petals of the Sahasrara. All of the nadis both emanate and terminate at this center.

Sahasrara is thought to be the abode of Shiva. It is also considered the place of the "guru within," known in the West as the Holy Guardian Angel. When Kundalini rises into the seventh chakra, all concepts of individuality are dissolved and the ego disappears into the bliss of Samadhi. The meditator becomes one with the entire universe; he has obtained occult power. In the yogic system he becomes a *Siddha* (one who possesses psychic power or the siddhis) but has risen above any desire other than to remain in the bliss of Samadhi.

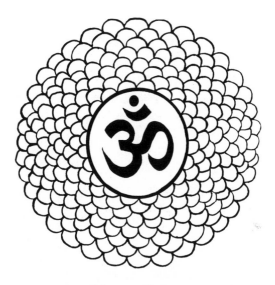

Sahasrara Chakra

A goddess or *shakti* called Paramatma is associated with this chakra. This is significant because in Vedic teachings, Paramatma is also considered the Supersoul. She is that which rises above the small "I" of conscious being. Paramatma is infinite and timeless, eternal, blissful, and wise. She may be compared with the Thelemic conception of Nuit.

THE ADVANTAGES OF CHAKRA WORK

Various Yoga practices can cause the sleeping Kundalini energy, lying coiled in the Muladhara chakra, to flow upward toward the higher centers. As the energy extends itself into the higher chakras, the magical consciousness will expand, and a person's attitude will change completely. Harish Johari, in his outstanding book *Chakras: Energy Centers of Transformation,* says that the feeling among people who have experienced or observed this change is consistently likened to a "new birth." He goes on to state:

> Maintaining the upward flow of energy then becomes the primary concern of such a person. The constant simultaneous practice of visualization and mantra japa [see page 76] helps the aspirant to maintain the flow of energy in higher centers and thus get beyond the tattwas and attain the nondual consciousness that liberates them from the illusory world of Maya.[9]

Try to learn as much about the chakras as possible. Mentally visualizing each one in detail is a great way to deepen meditation practices and to harmonize oneself with the chakra's corresponding energy. Exploration of the chakras, vibration of bija mantras, and adherence to the laws of *Dharma* or Righteousness through the practices of Yama and Niyama, are proven ways to maintain the flow of energy to the higher centers, expand consciousness, and ultimately enable a person to accomplish the Great Work. The practices described in the next section are the tools by which you may begin to accomplish this.

PART TWO

YOGA IN PRACTICE

CHAPTER FOUR

YAMA AND NIYAMA

Yama and Niyama build a person's character so
thoroughly that by sincerely practicing them one
ceases to be an animal, grows into a real human
being, and can even transform into the Lord.

SWAMI KRIPALU[14]

THE PRELIMINARY AIMS of Yoga are to keep the body healthy
and the mind balanced and serene. The behavioral observances detailed in the practice of Yama and Niyama are
designed to achieve these goals. I have listed the traditional
components of Yama and Niyama as passed down by gener-
ations of Yoga masters. They form a series of restrictions on
behavior (Yama) and directions for action (Niyama) whose
purpose is to help the Yogi achieve an acceptable degree of
serenity.

While I have wholeheartedly recommended the observances of physical exercise, proper diet, and meditation to
achieve those ends, it is up to you to decide exactly what diet,
exercise, and meditation practices are right for you. Similarly,
Yoga masters have proscribed and prescribed certain behavior for those who follow their teachings. Yet it is up to you to
experiment and decide what code of action is most effective
for your particular efforts in the Great Work.

The traditions and practices of Yama and Niyama were
developed in a totally different time and culture. While few of
us could even *comprehend* that complex, ancient society—
much less penetrate the depths of its religious philosophies
—these guidelines merit consideration.

The Magician is constantly creating his universe in as
conscious a manner as possible. It is important to be aware of

how things, people, and places affect you on a personal level: physically, mentally, and psychically. Also think about how your actions affect your state of mind. What impact do diet, exercise, meditation, and magical practices make on your life? What part do feelings play in your actions? Are you driven by jealousy, pride, joy, anger, inner resolve, or a combination of these many different things? The answers to such questions should matter to you.

It is very important to think for yourself and be brutally honest about your principles. You are responsible for setting your own codes of behavior and standards of living. Be ready to discard those things that don't work, even when it's a struggle. Decide what habits to persist in and cultivate. In *Magick: Book Four* Aleister Crowley summed up the practices of Yama and Niyama very practically, "The whole purpose of Yama and Niyama is to live so that no emotion or passion disturbs the mind." He was particularly anxious to divorce these principles of behavior from any type of superstition or cultural moral context. In the last sentence of the description of each Yama and Niyama, I have listed the traditional *siddhi*, or magical power associated with that behavior as given by Patanjali.

YAMA (Ethics)

Yama means "control" and its purpose is to eliminate things that distract or overly excite the mind. It is concerned with developing ethical principles. The practice of Yama applies to the outside world and how one interacts with others. Every man and every woman is a star, orbiting on his or her own trajectory: What is upsetting to one may not bother another. The goal of Yama is to create the lifestyle best suited to allow you to actually settle down and do your spiritual practices.

- *Ahimsa,* or nonviolence, is the first practice of Yama. Generally, this means not to harm any creature in any manner. On a deeper level, this yama implies that one should not even wish injury to others or (especially) to oneself. It is said that mastery of this yama renders all creatures harmless in one's presence.

- *Satya* means "honesty." It means both speaking the truth to the best of your knowledge as well as maintaining scrupulous self-honesty. Ultimately this yama invokes the power of truth-speaking; what faithful practitioners say will come to pass.

- *Asteya* is "nonstealing," and it refers to not taking what does not belong to you. This includes abstract concepts like status, love, and undeserved praise, as well as material objects. It also means not making unnecessary emotional demands on people or "stealing" their time and energy. Conversely, one should not allow another to steal from you, nor from others. It is said that individuals adept in Asteya will have whatever they need when they need it.

- *Brahmacharya* means "flowing with Brahma." This yama traditionally warns against overindulgence in the "pleasures of the senses." This yama cautions us to be conscious of the sexual choices we make. Be aware of the amount of energy you expend on sexual activity. Be honest and aware of how your sexuality affects your physical health, emotional state, energy level, and how it influences the choices you make in other aspects of your life. Careful practice of Brahmacharya gives good health, mental focus, and physical vigor.

- *Aparigraha* is the concept of noncovetousness or nongreed. On one level, this means letting go of attachments—such as to material objects, emotional crutches, and bad habits. As the process continues, there is a letting go of the very concept of the self: one's identity and physical body. One realizes there is something beyond the "veil of the senses." Mastery of this yama is said to give the ability to recall past incarnations.

NIYAMA (Practices, Observances)

In a very general sense, Niyama consists of religious actions or observances, as well as consistency and self-discipline in following one's spiritual practices. Unlike Yama, which deals with the outside, Niyama refers to inner discipline and responsibility. For some people, a Niyama observance may be as simple as meditation or solitary walks in the woods. Going to church, temple, or mosque is considered Niyama, as is practicing any consistent religious activity. Niyama is also seen as virtuous living, the cultivation of appropriate lifestyle choices, and the understanding, acceptance, and appreciation of those virtues in others.

- *Sauca* refers to cleanliness: both internal and external. This niyama not only directs people to keep their physical bodies properly functioning, but also refers to the necessity of inner clarity. The practices of Asana and Pranayama help to fulfill this niyama. It is said that mastery of Sauca leads to a holistic purity marked by an indifference to physical pleasure.
- *Samtosa* literally means happiness. It specifically refers to contentment and appreciation for what God has given: one's skills and basic personality. It includes being modest and "comfortable in one's

own skin." It is the ability to accept all things and beings as they are. Mastery of this niyama brings perpetual inner happiness and the awareness of bliss in all aspects of creation: every creature, every particle, every atom in the universe.

- *Tapas* means self-discipline and the cultivation of a healthy body. It means being aware of the body's needs: resting when appropriate, paying attention to proper posture, eating the right foods, and eating only when hungry. Practicing Tapas consistently brings the ability to remove unnecessary distractions and obtain control over personal prejudices. Mastery of this observance aids in attainment of various psychic powers (or siddhis).

- *Svadhyaya* is the fourth niyama. It counsels us to introspection. It is the echo of the ancient Western exhortation "know thyself." It is often tied to Mantra Yoga, however, it concerns all disciplines whose goal is oneness: Mantra Yoga, meditation, contemplation, and study. One objectively scrutinizes behavior, motivations, and desires when practicing Svadhyaya. Mastery brings the ability to communicate with Higher Intelligence.

- *Isvarapranidhana* means "to lay all actions at the feet of God." It is self-surrender, "pure will, unassuaged of purpose, delivered from the lust of result." The aspirant has done his or her best with the skills God has given. Now one offers the fruits of that labor in prayer. The outcome depends upon the Creator. Ultimately, this technique will allow communication with the Higher Power as one centers oneself in the Divine and allows God to do what he will.

CHAPTER FIVE

ASANA

Worship is possible in a seated posture

VYASA SUTRAS[15]

A*sana* means "posture." In the practice of Hatha Yoga, which deals with physical culture, stamina, and flexibility, asanas are the individual poses, like the Cobra or the Plow, that promote health. These types of asanas are usually part of a sequence of poses. For meditation, however, an asana is the physical position in which one chooses to work. An asana can be practiced sitting, standing, or lying down.

There is no person living on planet Earth who is not, at least on a subconscious level, in some degree of physical pain or discomfort. This is simply part of the human condition. The practice of Asana is designed to help one go beyond the interruptions of the body and to be able to sit perfectly still during meditation.

To perform Asana, simply take a firm and comfortable seat. However, the catch is that no position is truly comfortable to the average person! If you don't believe this or are not fully aware of this fact, try the following short experiment:

- Take a seat in any type of chair. Make sure to begin in a position that is comfortable.
- Take a look at the clock and note the time.
- Sit completely still.
- Let the mind wander. Make sure the body remains completely still.
- Note the sensations associated with the body: itching, tingling, burning. These phenomenon may

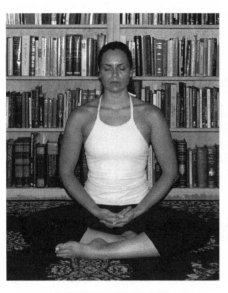

THE TAILOR'S POSE
(with hands in lap)

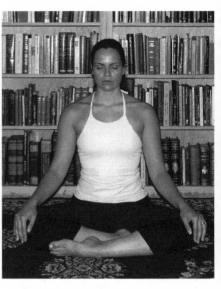

THE TAILOR'S POSE
(with hands on knees)

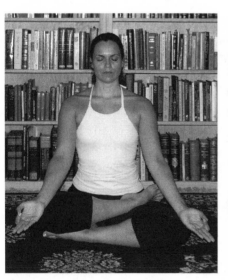

THE HALF LOTUS

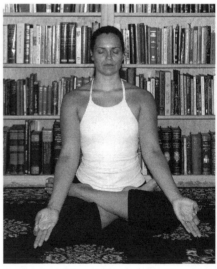

THE FULL LOTUS

start out mild but can advance to muscle cramps or spasms. One may be unable to suppress a cough, or the nose will start to run, or the eyes may tear up and become uncomfortable.

- Make a note of how many minutes into the experiment you were when these symptoms started, or when the body shifted of its own volition.

When I first tried this, my total time sitting still was about seven minutes. I was told that this was not too bad for a beginner.

When practicing Asana, it is important to pick a position and stick with it for a fair amount of time (like months or years) before switching to another position. This consistency gives an effective way to gauge progress. While Asana should be relatively comfortable, it should also be "firm," with a degree of natural muscular tension and skeletal rigidity. The spinal column should be straight. Two common, popular asanas are the following:

1. The Tailor's Pose (*Sukhasana*): this is also known as the "easy pose." Sit on the ground, a mat, or a cushion in a cross-legged position. Allow the hands to rest lightly on the knees, or be folded in the lap. The eyes should be nearly closed and cast downward as if looking at the lap. The spine should be straight but as relaxed as possible.

2. The Half Lotus (*Ardhapadmasana*): this is a variation of the lotus pose. Sit on the floor, the Yoga mat, or a cushion with the legs straight out in front. Bend the right leg, clasp the right foot in the hands and place it on top of the left thigh. Make sure the heel is as close to the navel as possible. Tuck the left foot under the right thigh. When using this position, alternate legs with each

practice so that both are stretched equally. (The Full Lotus, or *Padmasana,* is performed by placing each foot on top of the opposite thigh. It is considerably more difficult than the Half Lotus.)

In Liber E vel Exercitiorum,[16] Crowley recommends the following four poses:

1. The God: Sit in a straight-back chair. The spine should be straight, head up, knees together, eyes closed.
2. The Dragon: Kneel, let the buttocks rest on the heels. The toes should be turned back, the back and head are held straight, and the hands should rest on the thighs.
3. The Ibis: Stand, bend the left leg and grasp the left ankle with the right hand. Bring the left forefinger to the lips. Alternate practicing with the right ankle in the left hand.
4. The Thunderbolt: Sit, the left heel should press against the anus. The right foot is poised on its toes, the heel covering the phallus. Stretch the arms out over the knees. Keep the head erect and the spine vertical.

With the exception of the God pose, these positions may seem a bit intimidating. They may certainly seem more difficult than the Tailor's pose or the Half Lotus. However, the beauty of the asanas Crowley has described is that they confront physical limitations in a very big way. One who masters any of these poses will have overcome one of the most difficult hurdles on the road to enlightenment.

It is important to relax during Yoga practice, especially at the beginning and end. A good way to do this is to lie down in the Corpse pose. Lie face up on the mat with the

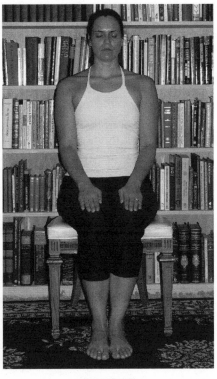

THE GOD

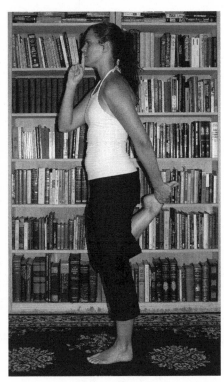

THE IBIS

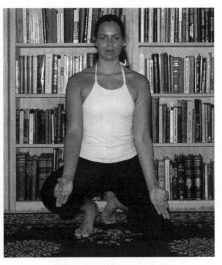

THE THUNDERBOLT

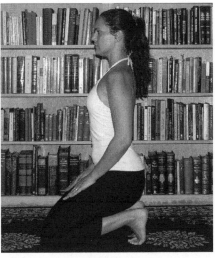

THE DRAGON

arms at approximately a forty-five degree angle from the body. The palms should be facing upward. Try to align the body as perfectly as possible. Legs should be straight, not bent, the lower legs and feet should be relaxed and rotated slightly outward. Let your muscles loosen and feel your whole body sink into the ground. Pay attention to the sensory organs: relax the tongue and the ears (both inner and outer), let your hands and fingers melt into the mat, and relax the eye muscles: you may imagine them looking at your heart or any other internal spot. Let the weight of the brain settle slowly to the back of the skull. Try to hold this pose for at least five minutes without falling asleep. When coming out of this asana, ease out of it as slowly as possible, in a relaxed manner. This is also an excellent way to begin astral projection practices.

The actual practice of Asana is similar to the experiment described earlier:

- Make sure to wear loose, comfortable clothing that will not interfere with the practice.
- After completing a preliminary banishing,[17] sit in the chosen position.
- Sit perfectly still for as long as possible.
- Make a note of what type of physical sensations are experienced and when they occurred during the exercise. Record them in your magical diary after finishing the exercise. If there is no pain at all, check to make sure the body has not shifted its position unconsciously.
- Unusual phenomenon may occur during these exercises. Write them down in detail immediately after practice so you can analyze them later.
- Strive to sit perfectly still for one hour without the slightest muscular disturbance: so still that if a

teacup full of water is balanced on the head, not a
single drop would spill.

You may wish to incorporate the use of *mudras*, or traditional hand gestures, while in Asana. There are times when
mudras serve to emphasize the purpose of a session. If you
decide to use a mudra, refrain from anything too complex.
One very simple mudra that is quite nice is the *abhaya*
mudra, also called the "gesture of fearlessness." It is depicted
in statuary and paintings of both Buddhist and Hindu deities.
Abhaya mudra symbolizes protection, serenity, and the elimination of fear. Simply raise the right hand to the chest at the
level of the heart with the palm facing out and fingers pointing toward the sky. The most common mudra for meditation
work is the *jnana* mudra. It represents knowledge. In jnana
mudra, the forefinger and thumb are touching. The remaining fingers are extended. If you wish to "open your awareness," allow the palms to face upwards. If the palms are
facing down, the effect is calming to the mind. The use of
mudras is entirely discretionary.

Despite its apparent simplicity, obtaining skill in the
practice of Asana is the cornerstone of all mystical exercises.
Proficiency in Asana is also important to a Magician performing "active" rituals. Whether pacing the boundaries of
the magical circle or spinning in ecstatic dance, the discipline
acquired through Asana is invaluable.

Perform Asana daily. The faithful use of Asana is one of
the best tools available to strengthen the Will. Remember to
write down the results in the magical diary, taking note of the
length of the practice, time of day, general health, mood, disposition, and so forth. Take time to analyze, at least briefly,
the phenomenon experienced during each session.

CHAPTER SIX

PRANAYAMA

*Yogis count life not by number of years but number of
breaths ... Every thought, every act of will, or motion
of muscles uses up this life force and in consequence
constant replenishing is necessary, which is possible
mainly through breathing alone.*

SWAMI VISHNUDEVANANDA[18]

THE PRACTICE OF PRANAYAMA involves the control of the
breath. The word *Prana* refers to a type of subtle energy that
animates every living thing. All activity is the result of Prana.
Physical energy is generated from Prana. Thought is considered the highest and most subtle form of Prana. As discussed
earlier, *Yama* means control. Thus, *Pranayama* refers to the
control of the life force. How does Pranayama relate to Magick? In the Western tradition, the Hebrew letter *Aleph* corre-
sponds with breath. Aleph and breath correspond with
Yetzirah, the Formative World. The number of Aleph is 1,
the mystic number of *Kether,* the *Sephira* from which all
other spheres emanate—the primary force. In the Tarot,
Aleph is symbolized by the airy, wandering Fool, poised on
the edge of the precipice, unwittingly and constantly creating
his reality.

In the classic modern text *Raja Yoga,* Swami Vivekananda writes that according to the Hindu philosophers, the
universe is composed of two different types of matter: *akasha*
and *prana*. Akasha is antimatter from which the elements
evolve. Air, liquids, and solids—the atmosphere, ocean, stars,
fish, plants, bugs, and humans—have all come from akasha.
Prana is the energy which creates akasha. At the end of their

cycle, every tangible element returns to akasha and all energy is absorbed back into prana. At the beginning of a creation cycle, prana stimulates akasha and universes are created. This cycle mirrors the concepts described in Crowley's *The Book of the Law* of the ever-expanding, ever-manifesting goddess of the night sky, Nuit (Akasha), and her consort, Hadit, the personification of focused, generative energy (prana): "In the sphere I am everywhere the centre, as she, the circumference, is nowhere found."

Breath is the physiological process associated with prana. The respiratory system moves prana throughout the body. The aim in Pranayama exercises is to control prana through manipulation of the breath.

The Kundalini is awakened and directed by Pranayama. For an aspirant of the Western path, the goal in Pranayama is to release as much Kundalini up the Shusumna as possible. Even the smallest amount of stimulation of the Kundalini force will affect the consciousness of the meditator.

Pranayama allows the mind and energies to focus together on one thing. When thought and breath are harmonized, a great deal of psychic power is created. The ability to focus the Will is enormously enhanced. Little else in the arsenal of the occultist can equal the power gained from the successful practice of Pranayama. It is a source of serenity and focus. It strengthens the subtle body and allows the adept to build the concentration necessary to complete other meditation exercises and magical work. Pranayama assists with astral projection or "rising on the planes." Dreams become more vivid and meaningful. Banishing rituals become more intense and powerful.

There are many different Pranayama exercises. Some are "even" cycles, where the length of inhalation and exhalation are the same. There are also "uneven" cycles, where the length of inhalation and exhalation vary. There is unified nostril breathing and alternate nostril breathing. There are *bandhas*, or "locks" which accompany more advanced methods designed to intensify the experience. There are also beautiful and elaborate rituals built around breathing exercises.

The three Pranayama exercises offered here are simple yet effective. To explore Pranayama in more depth, turn to the bibliography. The best method of learning advanced techniques in Pranayama is to find an experienced teacher.

During these exercises, relax into your asana. Remember the spine must remain as straight as possible. It is important to be relaxed and comfortable, yet alert. I do not recommend lying down. It is very easy to fall asleep or become torpid in that posture. Incidentally, it is best not to practice Pranayama or other forms of meditation after eating or when tired or ill.

Before beginning these exercises, spend some time learning to relax and simply focus on the breath. Time spent passively observing the breath and paying attention to its natural rhythm will help you learn to even it out during your actual Pranayama practices.

Using a metronome is an excellent way to help time the breath cycles. A metronome is also beneficial when working with a group. It helps to get everyone working at the same pace. Metronomes are quite affordable and may be purchased at any music store.

Pranayama: Exercise One
Unified Nostril Breathing

Sit in a comfortable position. Breathe in through the nose for eight counts. Hold the breath for eight counts. Breathe slowly out through the nose for eight counts. Hold the breath for eight counts. This is one cycle of Pranayama. Start with around twenty cycles, working up to sixty cycles or more. Focus solely on the breath. The mind will tend to wander; gently guide it back to an awareness of the breath. If inhaling or exhaling for eight counts is too difficult, start with a count of four and try to increase to eight-count cycles. One can extend this further: to ten-, twelve-, or even sixteen-count cycles. This exercise is very calming. It is also an excellent method to use with a group, especially prior to ritual.

Pranayama: Exercise Two
Alternate Nostril Breathing

Sit in a comfortable position. Using the ring and little fingers of the left hand, close the right nostril. Take a slow breath in through the left nostril to a count of eight. Hold the breath in for eight counts. Release the right nostril and block the left nostril with the left thumb. Breathe out slowly through the right nostril for eight counts. Hold the breath for eight counts. Repeat cycle beginning with opposite side (blocking the left nostril with the right hand, etc). Again, as in the first exercise, if you are having difficulty with eight counts, start with four and build up. This exercise is better suited to solitary work or with very small groups. It is quite relaxing. It is also useful to "blow out" negative energy prior to ritual.

Pranayama: Exercise Three
Kapalabhati

Sit in a comfortable position. Take two normal breaths, then inhale through the nose. Now exhale forcefully through the nose, while pulling in the abdomen. As soon as the exhalation is complete, relax the abdominal muscles. This will cause automatic inhalation. Repeat the cycle of automatic inhalation and forceful exhalation about fifteen times, keeping a steady rhythm and emphasizing the exhalation each time. Then inhale, exhale completely, inhale fully, and hold the breath for as long as comfortable. Slowly exhale. Repeat this sequence three times, working up to six sequences. It is easy to become dizzy during Kapalabhati, so it is important to take some slow deep breaths at the beginning and end of each cycle.

Unlike the first two breathing exercises, Kapalabhati is stimulating and energizing to all tissues in the body. It brings its own unique resonance into each of the chakras; successful practice will bring a feeling of joy. One will become very conscious of the spinal column, which will be invigorated and sensitive. This is an excellent exercise for use just prior to active magical work.

Proper practice of Kapalabhati makes one alert and vital. Additionally, Kapalabhati brings a physiological benefit. During Kapalabhati the nasal passages, sinuses, and lungs are cleared of excess mucus. It can help ease bronchial spasms. This practice is also said to free the body of great quantities of carbon dioxide.

CHAPTER SEVEN

MANTRA YOGA

Aum! tat savitur varenyam
Bhargo devasya dimahi
Dhiyo yo na pratyodayat.

O! let us strictly meditate on the
adorable light of that divine Savitri.
May she enlighten our minds!

GAYATRI MANTRA

ALEISTER CROWLEY DESCRIBES Mantra Yoga as being the parallel in speech to the control of the breath exercised in Pranayama. He further states that Mantra Yoga is the best way to time the breath during Pranayama. From these statements we can surmise that Pranayama and Mantra Yoga may be practiced at the same time.

Technically speaking, mantras are defined as "sacred words or phrases of spiritual significance and power." They are hymns which uplift the aspirant to the essence of their meaning. They both banish negativity and invoke the divine spark within the Magician or Yogi. In yogic tradition, the universe is constantly created through the medium of sound. Furthermore, Yogis believe that all sound, whether audible or inaudible issues from a supreme source known as *Shabda Brahman* ("supreme voice").

It is customary in India to invoke divine power, or the spirit of the teacher, when beginning any type of Yoga practice. This invocation assists the practitioner in setting his intention: defining the purpose of the work. It is also a way for the student to acknowledge the *source* of the power and wisdom he seeks to experience: the divine energies. Often the work itself is an invocation of a specific deity or archetype. The verbal incantations are recited as mantra.

When vocalized, mantras are known as *japa*, which means literally "muttering" or "whispering." A mantra can also be said silently, or *ajapa*. Some schools of thought maintain that while spoken or chanted mantra is effective, mantra is more potent when whispered. These schools further teach that ajapa mantras are even more effective than whispered mantras. In addition, it is believed that a mantra can be very effective when written on paper. This subcategory of ajapa mantra is know as *jikhita*.

Experiment with the various methods of Mantra Yoga. It is common to begin mantra meditation by slowly chanting the mantra aloud, then whispering it while steadily increasing the rate of repetition, and finally repeating the mantra silently for the remainder of the meditation, allowing it to reverberate rapidly through the mind. Properly performed, the mantra will be recited continuously, even during sleep. But this is a far more advanced stage.

So what exactly is the purpose of a mantra? The actual word is derived from the verb *man* which means "think" and the suffix *tra* which indicates conduciveness. Thus, mantra is conducive to thought: that is, it is a word or phrase that allows one to focus or intensify consciousness. Mantras cut through distracting thought patterns and purify intentions. Written records indicate that mantra has also been used for a variety of other reasons: from casting off demons, to controlling the behavior of others, obtaining magical powers, and praising the gods and goddesses.

In Liber O, Crowley recommends a specific method for uttering, or "vibrating" divine names during ritual and meditation. With some creativity, one might adapt this to the repetition of mantra. During the course of vibrating a god name, one completely absorbs the energy and quality of the name, breathing it in and letting it circulate through the entire body.

As soon as it becomes completely absorbed, the practitioner exhales and hurls it forth into the universe. At the end of the vibration, the exercise is sealed with the mudra of Harpocrates.[19]

Mantra Yoga practices become very intense when the mantra is visualized and absorbed in this manner. While repeating the mantra, let it circulate through your entire being, assimilating it on a cellular level while allowing it to penetrate all levels of the psyche and the highest levels of consciousness. At the end of the meditation session, project the mantra into the heavens. Finally, close with the sign of Harpocrates.

Another interesting exercise related to jikhita is to write out a chosen mantra and create an image around it. Hang the image in a place where you can see it frequently or use it as a type of yantra in meditation. It is a simplistic but effective approach to using an old technology in a creative way.

According to yogic tradition the best time to practice Mantra (and all types of Yoga) is *Brahma-Muhurta*, or "the hour of Brahma." While the exact time can vary somewhat from teacher to teacher, it is usually defined as either the hour of sunrise or the hour prior to sunrise. This may not be an appropriate time for all people. It is, however, beneficial to set aside a defined time for Yoga and magical practices. One key to success in both Magick and Yoga is consistency and determination.

The use of Mantra Yoga is widespread in Western esotericism. For example Dion Fortune found meditation and mantra to be important magical tools. In *Practical Occultism in Daily Life* she speaks of the use of a mantra as a means of invoking spiritual energy. She suggests that one should choose a mantra that expresses one's highest aspiration and say it over and over until "we find that it is beginning to take hold of us and repeat itself as a tune does that runs in one's head." She further explains:

When this occurs and we find that the mantram is repeating itself automatically, we know that it has gone down into the subconscious mind and is reappearing on the surface again. Now we are in a position to do the practical mental work because we have made subconscious contact with the Infinite, and even before any mental work is planned or done we shall be conscious of an inner change, a sense of wider life, of power, and freedom. As soon as this inner change begins to make itself felt we are in a position to deal magically with our environment, but not before.[20]

When choosing a mantra, try to find one that appeals to your understanding of the Great Work. For example, in Yoga "Om" (or Aum) is considered the universal mantra: the ultimate symbol of divine energy. One may wish to choose a more specific energy. If you are working within the Thelemic current, you may wish to use a phrase from a Thelemic text which has significance to you. For example, the following mantra taken from *The Book of the Law* is described by Crowley in *Magick: Book Four*, part 1 as "the holiest of all that are or can be."

A ka dua. Tuf ur biu. Bi aa chefu. Dudu ner af an nuteru.

(Unity uttermost showed!
    I adore the might of Thy breath,
Supreme and terrible God,
    Who makest the gods and death
To tremble before Thee: —
    I, I adore Thee!)[21]

Other useful mantras from various sources include:

- *Aum Mani Padme Hum!* (O! the Jewel in the Lotus! Amen!)
- *Qol: Hua Allahu achad; Allahu Assamad; lam yalid walam youlad; walam yakum lahu ufwan achad.* (Say: He is God alone! God the Eternal! He begets not and is not begotten! Nor is there like unto Him any one!)
- *Aum Tat Sat! Aum!* (O that Existent! O!)
- By thy name of Ra I invoke thee—Hawk of the Sun, the glorious one!
- There is no part of me that is not of the Gods.
- Let thy light crystallize itself in our blood, fulfilling us of resurrection.

The choices of mantra are almost limitless. The key rule to remember is to choose the mantra that represents the highest ideal. As Dion Fortune suggests, it is really better not to choose a mantra based on a specific need, but rather to choose the highest octave of the energy being invoked.

Working with Mantras

To begin the mantra practice, be seated in Asana. Systematically relax the muscles and straighten the spine, allowing it to lengthen from the sacral area of the pelvis. Relax the lumbar and thoracic areas of the spine, stretching into the cervical region of the neck. Let the hip bones settle into the ground. Release the facial muscles, letting the jaw slacken.

Focus now upon the breath. Observe and regularize the rhythms of the inhalations and exhalations. As the breathing steadies, start using a simple mantra. As an example, use

Aum as a way of connecting with the energy of the universe. Inhale and silently say, "Aum." Repeat the mantra aloud on the exhale. Note any discrepancies in the breathing and try to even out the sensations. Relax into the mantra. Let it go silent. You will be able to hear the sound of the mantra evenly in both the inhalation and the exhalation. The mantra should be a part of the breath, not separate from the breath.

After some practice with a monosyllabic mantra, one may wish to switch to a longer and more specific mantra. When using a more complicated mantra, again keep the focus on the evenness of breath. For example, when using the "A ka dua" mantra, the breath can be coordinated with the vocalization of the mantra. (Obviously, if one is saying the mantra aloud, this can only occur on the out breath). For instance:

(on the exhale) *A ka dua*
(on the exhale) *Tuf ur biu*
(on the exhale) *Bi aa chefu*
(on the exhale) *Dudu ner af*
(on the exhale) *an nuteru*

The "A ka dua" mantra may also be used as an ajapa mantra, in which case its verses may be recited silently during both the in breath and out breath.

Focus on the rhythm of the breath. Let it go in and out like the waves of the ocean, the breath/mantra slowly washing over and through you. If you lose focus, do not be disturbed; just turn the focus back to the mantra and the evenness of the breath. You may have chosen a mantra for a specific purpose, but while meditating, it's meaning becomes irrelevant. Should its purpose cross your mind, just guide your thoughts back to the tidal quality of the flow of the breath. If the meditation is being used in conjunction with ritual, there will be time for focus on the purpose later. Let everything go for now and concentrate on the mantra sound of the breathing.

It is a good idea to record the time spent in meditation in the magical diary. Deciding on a minimum time for meditation is an excellent discipline. Use a clock or a watch. Some people suggest setting a timer. Personally I feel it is jarring to be roused out of meditation by an alarm. On the other hand, perhaps one would not be distracted by thoughts about the time. Find what works best for you.

CHAPTER EIGHT

PRATYHARA

First hear, then understand,
and then, leaving all distractions,
shut your minds to outside influences
and devote yourselves to developing the truth
within you. There is a danger of frittering away
your energies by taking up an idea only for its
novelty and then giving it up for another that is
newer. Take one thing up and follow it, and see the
end of it, and before you have seen the end, do
not give it up. He who can become mad with
an idea, he alone sees the light. Those who
only take a nibble here and a nibble there will
never attain anything. They may titillate their
nerves for a moment, but there it will end.
They will be slaves in the hands of nature
and will never go beyond the senses.

SRI VIVEKANANDA[22]

EVERY DAY WE ARE DELUGED by an onslaught of ideas: political information, "reality TV," Sponge Bob, billboards, the local weather, radio "shock jocks," pop queens, "Michael Jackson," the pointless twaddle of eGroup commentators, podcasts and bloggers, sexual innuendo, the latest laundry detergent, and last evening's lotto winner. One message flickers off and is immediately replaced by a new inane directive. The assault is endless. We find ourselves in an involuntary trance, our minds whirling and endlessly repeating the daily sludge like rats running the boundaries in their cages.

The practice of Pratyhara is aimed at slowing and ultimately silencing the endless torrent of uninvited distractions: its purpose is to teach withdrawal and detachment from the senses. These techniques assist with developing introspection. Pratyhara helps to minimize and eliminate unwilled thoughts. It is a prerequisite for the more advanced practices of Dharana and Dhyana.

The process by which one approaches Pratyhara is deceptively simple. At first it may appear that Pratyhara is very easy, and that the mind is not really so cluttered after all. However, after a very short time, the continuous jumble of the "monkey mind," leaping from one distraction to another, will become conscious. It can be a tremendously frustrating experience. Only after a time of careful observation of these disturbances can a person slowly be able to detach from them. This is more difficult than stilling and detaching from the physical body during the practice of Asana. But it is an important part of discovering the way the mind works and, ultimately, in unlocking the door of the True Self.

To begin, sit in Asana and simply observe the thoughts that arise in consciousness. If at this point you try to stop them, the mind will become even more restless and more difficult to control. At the beginning just try to monitor the pattern of thoughts that come. You will notice that at times many different ideas pop into consciousness: some of them shockingly bizarre. Do not bother judging or analyzing them. Just continue to silently observe the ebb and flow of the mind. Eventually, after faithful, daily practice, the mind will become calmer and more disciplined. One will be approaching a more serene psychic environment. Eventually the mind will become perfectly controlled.

Traditionally, it is said that perfection of Pratyhara takes many years. Certainly it is advantageous for a Magician to practice it every day. Even at the beginning, the student benefits tremendously, as he begins to notice the thought patterns associated with his life. He is given the opportunity to change or discard those patterns, which are harmful or no longer useful. The ability to "clean house" is empowering: Life becomes fuller and more meaningful when the excess clutter of obsolete thoughts and ideas is swept away. While discussing emptying the mind, it is wise to briefly mention the dangers of hypnosis. It is a fairly common practice today to employ hypnosis as a tool to empty and still the mind. Indeed, on the surface, hypnosis would be a very practical way to approach the serenity one aims for in Pratyhara exercises. In fact, it may not be such a bad thing for a person with no interest in mysticism or the occult arts. However, a Magician or mystic must remember that to allow the mind to be controlled by another person through hypnotic suggestion introduces the significant danger that one's own control is weakened. Even when employing the services of a certified hypnotherapist, something as banal as "guided imagery" can be detrimental if one allows another person to plant these images in the mind. Magicians must strive to develop the strongest mind possible. Swami Vivekananda found hypnotherapy reprehensible and felt that it led to the mind's ruin. There is nothing a hypnotist can do for you that you cannot accomplish alone. One builds strength by doing one's own work.

On the other hand, the practice of imagery may be used as a tool to help prepare the mind for Pratyhara as well as other mystical practices. There are several good books available that offer excellent ideas for *creating your own* imagery. Some of these are listed in the bibliography.

In my opinion, the most effective instruction available to prepare oneself for the practice of Pratyhara remains Aleister Crowley's Liber III vel Jugorum. On the surface, Liber Jugorum makes one hyperconscious of every move, every word, and every thought one generates. This state of self-consciousness is the exact opposite of the goal of Pratyhara. However, the purpose of Liber Jugorum is to make a person aware of the unconscious and mechanistic nature of words, actions, and thoughts. This knowledge enables one to stop the endless repetition of distracting thoughts: which *is* the goal of Pratyhara.

This clarity can also reveal underlying unconscious motivations behind behaviors. Crowley's instructions in Liber Jugorum state that the aspirant should, with each transgression, make a cut in his forearm with a razor blade. This may not be a viable option for many people. I have had good results using a thick, tight rubber band around the wrist. With each transgression, a sound, welt-raising *thwack* did the trick! I had a swollen arm as I persisted, but was able to avoid too many inquiries from coworkers and family. My Pratyhara practices improved rapidly during that period.

Here are the exercises, extracted from Liber III vel Jugorum, for monitoring and control of words, actions, and thoughts.

FOR SPEECH:

Here are practices. Each may last for a week or more.

1. Avoid using some common word, such as "and" or "the" or "but"; use a paraphrase.

2. Avoid using some letter of the alphabet, such as "t" or "s" or "m"; use a paraphrase.

3. Avoid using the pronouns and adjectives of the first person; use a paraphrase.

Of thine own ingenium devise others.

FOR ACTION:

Here are practices. Each may last for a week or more.

1. Avoid lifting the left arm above the waist.

2. Avoid crossing the legs.

Of thine own ingenium devise others.

FOR THOUGHT:

Here are practices. Each may last for a week or more.

1. Avoid thinking of a definite subject and all things connected with it, and let that subject be one which commonly occupies much of thy thought, being frequently stimulated by sense-perceptions or the conversation of others.

2. By some device, such as the changing of thy ring from one finger to another, create in thyself two personalities, the thoughts of one being within entirely different limits from that of the other, the common ground being the necessities of life.

Of thine own ingenium devise others.[23]

Pratyhara in Practice

A classical approach to the actual practice of Pratyhara meditation is to employ the *Sanmukhi* mudra in which the sensory organs of the head are covered with the hands, physically blocking out external stimuli. The thumbs gently press into the ears, while the remaining fingers cover the eyes, nose, and mouth. Relax the entire face and keep the fingers lightly placed and sensitive. Try to keep an even pressure. Imagine each sense as blank and still. Begin by utilizing this mudra for several minutes only. After releasing the hands, continue sitting in your asana. Try to maintain the stillness as long as possible. However, do not actively fight the reemergence of sensory awareness and thoughts: to do so defeats the purpose of the practice. It is especially important not to practice with the Sanmukhi mudra if you have an ear, eye, or sinus infection.

It is through Pratyhara that the subtle body gathers power and opens itself to divine inspiration. Pratyhara stimulates awareness of one's role within the flow of the universe. It is an essential step toward the ultimate goal of Western occultism: the Knowledge and Conversation of the Holy Guardian Angel.

CHAPTER NINE

SAMYAMA: ADVANCED YOGA PRACTICES
Dharana, Dhyana, and Samadhi

*I am he, as you are he, as you are me,
and we are all together!*

THE BEATLES

MEDITATION IS THE KEY TO OCCULT POWER. Within the system of Yoga, meditation is considered the key to obtaining enlightenment. *Samyama* is the act or "flow" of meditation. In the classical sense, Samyama refers to three different components of meditation.

1. Dharana: a single-pointed focus upon an object
2. Dhyana: the ability to see the underlying truth of the object of meditation
3. Samadhi: the absorption or union of the ego and the object of meditation

It is important to understand that these remaining three "limbs" of Ashtanga Yoga are interdependent and interrelated. It is impossible to experience Dhyana without first passing through Dharana. It is common to move between states of Samadhi and Dhyana within a single meditation session; these levels of consciousness are very close to one another and the delineation between the two is blurred at best. It is also possible to move into Samadhi spontaneously while practicing Dharana.

In Samyama, the mind is gently turned from the outward senses into the inner spheres, giving the individual a new reference point. One becomes intimately aware of the "bigger picture" and arouses energy and levels of consciousness previously unavailable. These psychic events redefine daily life in several different ways:

- Creativity and intuition are enhanced.
- Stress levels are lowered.
- Because consciousness is raised, the entire "personality" can change, regrouping around a higher center.
- Wisdom increases through enhanced insight.

Samyama takes the Magician to an entirely different level. One's very concepts of Magick and occult power evolve as perspective is elevated.

Dharana, Dhyana, and Samadhi do not come easily: well, they certainly don't to me! While the actual practice seems simple enough, doing Yoga on a regular basis is hard work. Sitting in stillness waiting for a connection with the universe to create itself is very difficult for the average esotericist. It is so much easier to construct magical circles, chant incantations, and dance around while summoning the forces of the universe to our beck and call!

Why bother with this Samyama business? Because it is only here that the *true* magical work begins. The more we give ourselves over to the stillness and silence, the easier it is to hear the voice of the Holy Guardian Angel.

The instructions for Dharana, Dhyana, and Samadhi are relatively straightforward and short because the actual method of meditation practice is uncomplicated. I do not seek to bog you down with unnecessary theory. Practice is the key.

The breeze at dawn has secrets to tell you.
> Don't go back to sleep.
You must ask for what you really want.
> Don't go back to sleep.
People are going back and forth across the doorsill
> where the two worlds touch.
The door is round and open.
> Don't go back to sleep.

RUMI[24]

Dharana

. . . the stopping off decisively our miscellaneous activity, and concentrating our force on one or a few points; as the gardener, by severe pruning, forces the sap of the tree into one or two vigorous limbs, instead of suffering it to spindle into a sheaf of twigs.

RALPH WALDO EMERSON[25]

Dharana is the sixth limb of Ashtanga Yoga. In Sanskrit, the prefix "*Dhr*" means "to hold." Simply put, Dharana is the restraint of conscious thought to one object. This concentration is not forced, like when an analyst concentrates on working out a difficult problem in a computer program. The concentration experienced in Dharana is more passive and occurs in a state of relaxed awareness. Take the example of pouring a large amount of sand into a receptacle with several smaller compartments. If each compartment were the same size, the sand would flow into all the compartments at an equal rate. However, if one of the compartments was wider and deeper than the others, a greater amount of sand would flow more rapidly into that compartment. This is basically what happens during the practice of Dharana. The meditator creates a deeper compartment that allows the mind to flow more rapidly in that one particular direction.

The point of Dharana is to focus the mind on a particular object. It is good to begin the practice by focusing on a simple yantra. In addition to being used as a central point in meditation, yantras may also be used for worship and protection. Yantras can be very complex, but for the purposes of this exercise, should be simple. A single black point in the midst of a white background is an appropriate choice. When comfortable working with external objects, try turning the attention inward. One may find one of these inner points of focus helpful:

- Roll the eyes upward and concentrate on a spot in the center of the forehead.
- Roll the eyes downward as if gazing at the navel.
- Roll the eyes forward as if looking at the nose.

The general idea is to keep the mind from wandering and to deliberately hold it on a particular, relatively static object. These simple exercises are believed to go a long way toward purifying the Body of Light.

Once you feel you've attained some success with the exercises above, you may wish to advance these simple instructions a little bit. Vivekananda points out that it is useful to engage the imagination. For example, bring the attention to the base of the throat. Feel only the throat and no other part of the body. Imagine the Vishuddha chakra in its place at the base of the throat, pulsing and glowing with radiant light. Focus the mind in that place. These instructions can be applied to any place on the body. These exercises can also uncover a great potential for inner healing.

Begin the practices slowly. Aleister Crowley recommends that the student start with just a minute or two, keeping track of breaks in concentration, and gradually lengthening the time. Do not become discouraged if you notice more breaks in concentration as you continue. This is probably due to the fact that you are becoming a better observer. The breaks will decrease in time. Just remember that the mind is like a Labrador puppy: it likes to roam around everywhere and frequently loses itself! As with other Yoga practices, when the mind wanders, gently guide it back to where it belongs.

Crowley outlines a very simple method of practicing Dharana in Liber E, part 5. It is extracted here for your reference.

DHARANA: CONTROL OF THOUGHT

1. Constrain the mind to concentrate itself upon a single simple object imagined.

   The five tattwas are useful for this purpose; they are: a black oval; a blue disk; a silver crescent; a yellow square; a red triangle.
2. Proceed to combinations of simple objects; e.g. a black oval within a yellow square, and so on.
3. Proceed to simple moving objects, such as a pendulum swinging, a wheel revolving, etc. Avoid living objects.
4. Proceed to combinations of moving objects, e.g. a piston rising and falling while a pendulum is swinging. The relation between the two movements should be varied in different experiments.

   Or even a system of flywheels, eccentrics, and governor.
5. During these practices the mind must be absolutely confined to the object determined upon; no other thought must be allowed to intrude upon

the consciousness. The moving systems must be regular and harmonious.

6. Note carefully the duration of the experiments, the number and nature of the intruding thoughts, the tendency of the object itself to depart from the course laid out for it, and any other phenomena which may present themselves. Avoid overstrain; this is very important.

7. Proceed to imagine living objects; as a man, preferably some man known to, and respected by, yourself.

8. In the intervals of these experiments you may try to imagine the objects of the other senses, and to concentrate upon them.

    For example, try to imagine the taste of chocolate, the smell of roses, the feeling of velvet, the sound of a waterfall, or the ticking of a watch.

9. Endeavor finally to shut out all objects of any of the senses, and prevent all thoughts arising in your mind.... [26]

Patanjali recommends the student commence the practice of Dharana while repeating the Aum mantra and gazing at its symbol. You may start by placing an image of the word Aum at eye level. It should be positioned so it is easy to see. The recitation of the mantra should be relaxed and easy but deliberate. Do not strain the vocal cords. Thus one will see the image with the eyes, chant the word with the tongue, and hear the mantra with the ears. Three of the five sensory organs are centering on the mantra, which encourages the mind to fix itself on Aum as well. (One could certainly add rosary-type beads for touch and a specially chosen incense for smell).

When comfort is achieved, the mind relaxed, and the attention is on the mantra, stop pronouncing it aloud and close

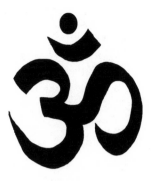

AUM Symbol

the eyes. Focus on the memories of Aum as experienced by the eyes, tongue, and ears. When the experience transcends the senses and is accomplished unbroken in the mind, it is considered "true" Dharana.

Success in Dharana requires steady, regular practice and like Pratyhara, it takes time to progress. Do not be discouraged. Working with Dharana brings a feeling of peace, increases objectivity, broadens perspective, and improves physical health.

During these Yoga practices, it is important to be aware of one's surroundings and the company one keeps. The meditation space should be as pleasant as possible, clean and free of cold or warm air drafts, lights that are too bright, or excess noise. The area should be free of strong smells: whether from food, pungent incense, or laundry. One should take pleasure in the meditation space.

During periods of intense practice, one should limit social contact as much as possible. Ideally, one should have a dedicated space devoted solely to Magick or meditation. If this is not feasible, make sure only positive people enter your sphere. Those who are cynical, clingy, hostile, or derisive should not be allowed in the home, especially if meditation takes place in an "open" area of the home.

Magical retreats are also useful. These can be as simple as a weekend spent in solitary meditation. Warn family and friends, refuse to answer the door, let the message machine pick up the phone, forget about the Internet. One will emerge from such an experience refreshed and invigorated.

Dhyana

The normal mind is a candle in a darkened room. Throw open the shutters, and the sunlight makes the flame invisible. That is a fair image of Dhyana.

ALEISTER CROWLEY[27]

Dhyana is perfect contemplation. In Dhyana we have moved beyond the single-pointed focus of Dharana into the consciousness of cosmic truth. It is worship, but only in the passive, reflective sense. It is religious, but only in a profoundly abstract way. In Dharana, one is a single-pointed observer; in Dhyana one understands and unveils the true nature of the object being contemplated. Dhyana cannot be practiced, per se. A person can, however, create an appropriate environment for it to occur. In the relative mental silence achieved by the work of Pratyhara, a more favorable environment for Dharana is achieved. With repeated efforts of this type, one may flow naturally into Dhyana.

Dhyana is similar to Samadhi. Like Samadhi, Dhyana involves an abolition of space, time, and causality. It has been said that duality dissolves and the veils of perception around the object or concept being contemplated are pierced. Consciousness becomes aligned with the universe and we draw pure insights between words, their meanings, the ideas generated by the words, as well as between ideas in our minds, the means of perception, and the objects perceived. Most importantly, one realizes these concepts are connected, and that they are all single, united, and equal in the continuum of the universe.

In Dhyana, the mind fully grasps the differences between itself and the object of meditation. This is important as there must be a clear concept of what each is in order to understand the similarities and to fully identify with the object of contemplation. In this sense, being in a state of Dhyana means seeing things as they truly are, understanding what they truly are, and what their relation to ourselves actually is. The mantras and yantras become passwords and beacons into the inner realms. The interior space is like an endlessly twisting maze that shall be explored and examined in order to find the goal. The intellect falls away in the slipstream of the subconscious mind and the symbols draw us deeper into our true selves and the true nature of existence. The intellect perceives the symbols on an abstract level and during deep meditation the meaning of the yantras and mantras become pure, explicit, and profound.

Again, Dharana, Dhyana, and Samadhi are inextricably intertwined. There are no specific exercises for Dhyana. When meditation practices advance, a connection will form between the Magician or Yogi and the object of meditation. This connection cannot be forced, but with proper practice will occur naturally.

As an example, let us expand the experiment from the section on Dharana. Assume one has chosen to explore the nature of the Muladhara chakra. The appropriate yantra has been drawn out and painted. It has been placed at eye level as one sits in Asana.

Focus the eyes on the Muladhara yantra. Repeat the Muladhara's bija mantra, *Lang*, aloud. Hear this sound coming from the Muladhara chakra. Experience it as all-encompassing, resonating through the entire being. Feel the Muladhara chakra itself vibrate. Let the vibration spread to the other chakras. Continue to repeat the mantra. While chanting, look at the yantra and imagine that it is the actual Muladhara chakra, and that it is also the mantra one hears repeating itself within the psyche. Let the mantra run silent. Know that the deity, the chakra, the yantra, the colors, the mantra, and the meditator are one. Now visualize the yantra in the area of the pineal gland, at the Ajna chakra. Continue to repeat the bija mantra silently.

In Dharana, the mind is single pointed, flowing in only one direction. In Dhyana, one connects with the object, communicates with it, and identifies with it. The realization arises that everything, the entire universe, is created of the same fabric. As consciousness expands the ego shrinks, making room for direct experience of the universal energy. The loss of ego is the most important point of Dhyana.

Samadhi

This is the creation of the world, that the pain of division is as nothing, and the joy of dissolution all.

THE BOOK OF THE LAW

What is Samadhi? It is a state in which the practitioner becomes one with the object of meditation, a supreme union with spiritual supraconsciousness, and the last stage of Ashtanga Yoga.

Samadhi literally means "to bring together, to merge." So, does this mean that Samadhi is what occurs when a person in meditation becomes so absorbed in something he loses consciousness of everything else? This is almost correct. In

Samadhi an individual's personal identity: name, profession, family history, social security number, driver's license photo, etc. completely disappears. Nothing separates him from the objective universe; the veils of mundane perception are torn asunder. Both his nature and the nature of the object on which he has been meditating merge into the universal existence. As a result of this merging, consciousness is elevated to perceive the divine nature of all existence, and union with the Absolute is achieved.

Samadhi is a state which cannot be expressed. It is above the mind's thought processes. Speech and intellect are of no use at this level. Samadhi is a state of complete and utter calmness in which consciousness is unwavering.

During Samadhi, it is said that one realizes what it means to be at one with the universe, no different than any object in the cosmos. This awareness sets one free and the soul can realize its true nature. A person becomes aware that his very nature is Brahman. The conscious mind rises into the empyrean heights from which it first emerged. The final stage of Samadhi ends at the very instant the soul is freed. This complete freedom of an individual soul moves it beyond all time and place. Once freed, it does not return to its confinement.

Samadhi is a mysterious state. Some Yogis mistakenly think Samadhi must involve loss of consciousness, cessation of breath or heartbeat, and other climactic phenomena. Because of this, many Yogis practice rigorous types of Pranayama aimed at slowing and stopping their breath. These disciplines are very difficult for most people, so even the most devoted students inevitably become frustrated and discouraged, feeling that they are not making sufficient progress. These students are mistaking physical states for spiritual states and conditions.

Swami Sivananda wrote regarding Samadhi: "Here the mind becomes identified with the object of meditation; the meditator and the meditated, thinker and thought become one in perfect absorption of the mind."

There are various stages of Samadhi, depending upon whether one is identified with the object while yet conscious of the object, or whether one has transcended the object of meditation and is resting in the experience of being without conceptual support.

Despite its popular description as an extremely profound metaphysical occurrence, Samadhi is considered to be mankind's natural spiritual state. The Yoga Sutras imply that the true self is "actionless" and always in Samadhi. The conditions of external existence force us out of our natural state of awareness. We forget our divine origins. To regain this awareness, the mystic begins to turn back toward the Self, toward the True Will.

When a person begins to understand on a spiritual, emotional, or intellectual level that he or she is, in fact, one with the universe, life is perceived differently. Without engaging in New Age jargon, it is clear that with the recognition of divinity comes the awareness that each person truly does create his or her own universe. If anything is holding a person back from attaining Samadhi, it is that person's own negative thoughts and misconceptions. This is one of the reasons gurus advise their followers to cultivate joy and to push negative thoughts aside. The theory is that constantly dwelling on the bad things that happen causes more bad things to happen. Conversely, focusing on the good things in life and positive possibilities will allow one's experiences to grow more positive. This is not to say that one should not be a realist, taking the necessary precautions to ensure physical, psychic, and emotional safety. Precaution and foresight are positive traits. Cultivating the qualities of discernment and deliberate action is a basic part of the purification process.

To repeat, Dhyana and Samadhi cannot be "practiced." One cannot just sit in his Asana and decide he is going to "do Dhyana," like he would do a Tree pose. All one can do is create a favorable state of mind conducive to the experience of Samyama. For example, there are Asana postures and types of Pranayama that create conditions favorable for the experience of Samyama. The Yoga Sutras say that in order to experience Dharana and Dhyana, the mind must first be relaxed, open, and in a particular psychic state. Allow the many things that are going on in the mind to settle so that it becomes quiet.

Some people describe Samadhi as a state of being very aware of things, but not possessing a point of view about any part of the experience. During Samadhi a person is aware of many different perspectives and facets of reality, but remains detached from any of them.

Samadhi is a state of mind in which one's experiences of family, culture, education, and history no longer influence perception. Samadhi is the direct experience of reality. Each of us has experienced Samadhi for very brief periods of time. It may happen during an intense sexual experience; it may happen diving under ocean waves. Magicians may experience it during ritual. Samadhi is that state in which one is intimately aware, with the simple certainty of a young child, of the essential unity of all creation.

Ultimately, what does exploration of Yoga hold for a student of the occult? How does Samadhi correlate to life? So much of mundane life is repetition: one goes to work, does the laundry, weeds the garden, cooks dinner, and pays the bills. Why should one add the repetitive discipline of Yoga and Magick, patiently doing the practices: banishing, stretching, Pranayama? Why does one feel compelled to keep searching for the higher ground when it seems that these ancient concepts, like Samadhi, appear to be so outside the flow of modern life?

While Samadhi may seem to have nothing to do with our existence or culture, in truth, it is the most important thing that could ever happen to us. Within the concept of Samadhi lies the seed of hope. Patanjali stated that Samadhi was an experience that anyone is capable of at any time in their lives. Acceptance of Patanjali's belief is an affirmation of the inherent divinity in each of us. We all have the potential to become fully conscious beings. Yoga and Magick are necessary steps on the path to reality. The experience of Samadhi marks the actual beginning of the Great Work. The Magician is able to experience communication with his Angel and to take the first step on his journey to fulfill the True Will.

Best of luck to all of you in your experiences.

> Out beyond ideas of wrong doing and right doing,
>   there is a field. I'll meet you there.
> When the soul lies down in that grass,
>   the world is too full to talk about.
> Ideas, language, even the phrase *each other*
>   doesn't make any sense.
>
> RUMI[28]

APPENDIX ONE

THE MIDDLE PILLAR

CHAKRAS AND THE BODY OF LIGHT

AN EXCELLENT WAY to incorporate your knowledge of the chakras with the practices of Asana, Pranayama, Mantra Yoga, and Pratyhara is the Middle Pillar exercise. (The Tree of Life is composed of ten spheres and twenty-two paths arranged in three pillars as illustrated on the next page.) Although the Middle Pillar exercise is a wonderful practice for the Magician of any level of development, it is an especially valuable tool for the beginner. It gives an appropriate method of becoming aware of and working with magical energy. Regular practice purifies the nadis and brings a profound awareness of the chakras. In my experience, this exercise is a great way to build energy prior to ritual and an excellent tool for building god-forms.

Dr. Israel Regardie introduced the Middle Pillar ritual to the modern Western occult tradition. He stated in *The Complete Golden Dawn System of Magic* that he could find no references to the technique in the original Golden Dawn papers, but was able to trace its origin to Dr. Felkin of the Stella Matutina (a later Golden Dawn offshoot that included Dion Fortune among its members). He says that Dr. Felkin described the ritual in an undeveloped form in one of the Order's grade papers. Regardie then perfected and popularized it in *The Middle Pillar, The Art of True Healing, The Complete Golden Dawn System of Magic,* and *The Foundations of Practical Magic.*

The ritual proceeds as follows: Begin (as always) by attuning the aura and consecrating the psychic space with the

THE TREE OF LIFE

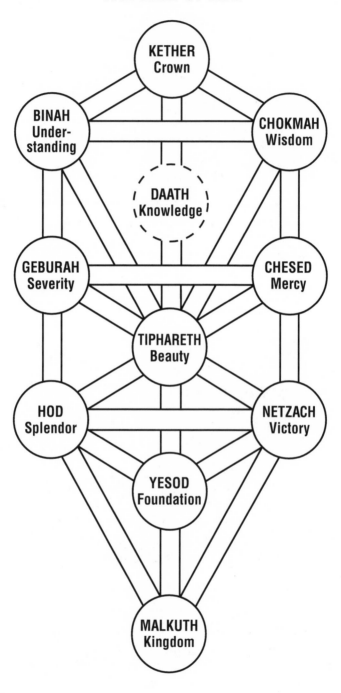

Lesser Banishing Ritual of the Pentagram (or a similar ritual such as the Star Ruby).

Engage in conscious relaxation using deep breathing and Yoga postures to free the body of its deeper stresses and strains.

Imagine a ball of scintillating white light (considerably larger than a grapefruit and considerably smaller than a basketball) coalescing both above and interpenetrating with the top of the skull (the Sahasrara chakra or Kether position). Vibrate the Divine Name EHIEH (eh-hee-yeh) several times, while the sphere of light grows brighter and more vibrant. Regardie suggests at least five minutes.

When the visualization is firmly established, allow the energy to descend slowly through the head and face, bathing and rejuvenating oneself, until it comes to the throat. Here the light coalesces in the Vishuddha chakra or Daath position and is of a pale purple or lavender color. Vibrate the name YHVH ELOHIM (yeh-ho-vah el-o-heem) until comfortable with the level of concentration and ready to go on.

Allow the energy to descend through the upper chest region with the same purifying and flowing movement until it comes to the heart or Tiphareth region, being the Anahatta chakra. Vibrate the name YHVH ELOAH VA DAATH, (yeh-ho-vah el-o-ah vah-daath) while visualizing a sphere of golden light growing richer and brighter.

Then take the energy through the solar plexus and stomach, down to the base of the trunk at the genital region, where it meets a sphere of deepest rich purple at the Yesod position or Svadisthana chakra. Here vibrate the name SHADDAI EL CHAI (sha-dai el chai). (There is no equivalent in English to the Hebrew "CH" sound; it is a guttural sound, similar to clearing the throat.)

The energy now descends through the thighs, knees, and shins until it coalesces at the feet in the Malkuth position. Here the crossover to the chakra system is more tenuous although, in my opinion, this position is analogous to the Muladhara chakra. This is particularly evident if one performs the ritual in a seated, cross-legged position. The Malkuth sphere is visualized as deepest vibrating black in color. The Divine Name is ADONAI HA-ARETZ (pronounced as spelled).

Now that the Middle Pillar has been formulated, one visualizes the energy rising through the body, passing upward through the spheres. It ascends from the black sphere at the feet, through the legs to the purple sphere at the genitals, through the stomach and solar plexus to the golden sphere at the heart, through the chest to the lavender sphere at the throat, and up through the face to the white sphere at the crown of the head. Here one concentrates on the glowing white brilliance and begins the work of the three Circulations.

The energy is first visualized as descending down and outward from the crown sphere, along the left side of the body during the out-breath, until it reaches the left foot. Then it crosses over to the right foot and ascends, on the in-breath, until it returns to the crown chakra at the completion of the in-breath. This should be done numerous times until one can feel a flowing motion, timed to the breathing, which is most rejuvenating.

Continue on to the second circulation. It also begins at the crown sphere and goes forward and down the front of the body, on the out-breath, until it reaches the feet. Then, on the in-breath, the energy proceeds up and around the back of the body, until it returns to the sphere of white brilliance at the crown of the head on the completion of the in-breath. Continue to circulate the light in this manner until it is felt as real (which is easier than it may sound).

Finally, the last circulation is performed. With the energy at the crown, the light is visualized as descending again through the Middle Pillar, until it reaches the Malkuth sphere at the feet. From here, it is circulated up and through the body to the crown on the in-breath. When it reaches the crown, it is imagined as "fountaining" at the completion of the in-breath, before the out-breath begins. The fountaining energy goes up and out through the crown and then down and around the body during the out-breath until it reaches the feet when the out-breath is complete. It is raised again with the in-breath, and the cycle of raising, fountaining, and descending continues until the ritual is closed.

* * *

Dr. Regardie insisted on the importance of practicing the circulations, even in the initial stages of learning the ritual.

There are adaptations possible for the Divine Names of the spheres more appropriate to Thelemic theology. These Words of Power were arrived at by early members of TAHUTI Lodge through a study of Crowley's Liber V vel Reguli in *Magick in Theory and Practice*.

At Kether one may substitute the Divine Name NUIT.

At Daath, the Name AIWASS.

At Tiphareth, vibrate RA-HOOR-KHUIT.

At Yesod, HADIT.

At Malkuth, the conjoined Name BABALON-THERION.

APPENDIX TWO

SOLAR WORKINGS

Salutation to the Sun &
Liber Resh vel Helios

IN THE EASTERN TRADITIONS, the sun is connected with general health and longevity. In Western occultism, it is connected with the sphere of Tiphareth, the heart center, which also rules health and healing. The yogic Salutation to the Sun (*Soorya Namaskar*) is a foundation practice of Hatha Yoga. This simple sequence of stretching exercises is something the occult practitioner can use for an infinite variety of purposes. The Sun Salutation is a perfect way to precede Pranayama and meditation. It is also a great way to "loosen up" before beginning any magical ritual. The body, heart, and lungs will be functioning optimally and the mind will be relaxed and ready to focus on the work at hand.

In the Thelemic tradition, one of the key practices is Liber Resh, the Adorations of the Sun. It is performed four times daily: at dawn, noon, sunset, and midnight. Optimally the Solar Adorations should be followed by meditation. The Adorations of Liber Resh and the yogic Sun Salutations are a perfect combination of practices, a marriage of East and West, Yoga and Magick.

Although the Sun Salutation is simple, it can be challenging for the beginner. It is important to remember that the beauty of Hatha Yoga is the gradual nature of the physical exercise. People of varying degrees of flexibility and fitness can improve their health through continued practice. With practice, comes progress.

There are twelve different positions that make up Soorya Namaskar; each one stretches different muscle groups. The different movements manipulate the vertebral column in different ways, so the spine and spinal muscles get a complete stretch. During the forward-bending sequences, the abdomen contracts, enabling deep exhalation. Conversely, during the backward-bending poses, the chest expands and deep breathing transpires naturally.

For beginners, it is a good idea to start with (or work toward) six repetitions of the cycle. If doing more than one set at a time, alternate leading with right and left legs (see steps 4 and 9). For example, lead with the right leg in the first set then the left leg in the second set.

SALUTATION TO THE SUN

1. Face the sun and stand straight with your arms at your side. The legs should be straight with the feet together. Exhale and bring the palms together at the level of the heart.
2. Inhale, raising your arms over your head. Bend backward.
3. Exhale and bend forward, touching the floor and bringing the hands in line with the feet. Touch the knees with your head. (You may bend your knees if you need to). Keep your chin tucked in to your chest. After a little practice you should be able to reach your knees with no problem.
4. Inhale and take a big step backward with your right leg. Bend the right knee to the floor and stretch the head up and back. Only the right foot changes position in this pose; the left foot and hands remain where they are (the left knee should be between the hands).
5. Hold the breath. Move the left leg back to the right leg, keeping feet together, knees and hips aligned. Rest on your hands, keeping your arms

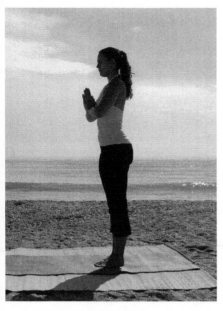

POSITION 1

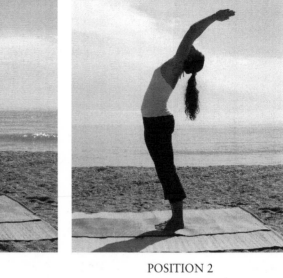

POSITION 2

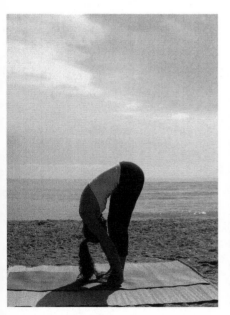

POSITION 3

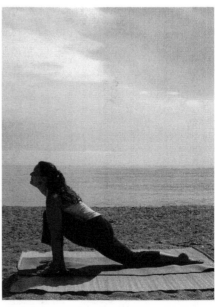

POSITION 4

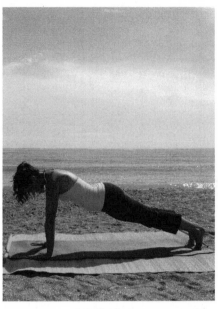

POSITION 5

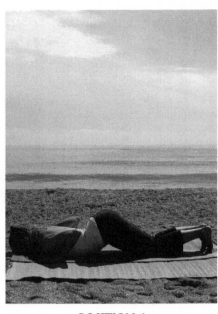

POSITION 6

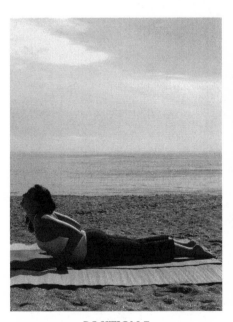

POSITION 7

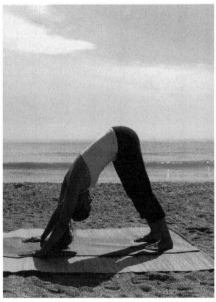

POSITION 8

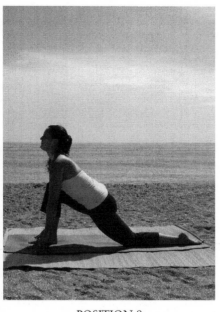

POSITION 9

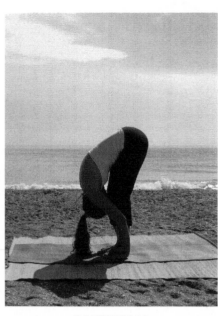

POSITION 10

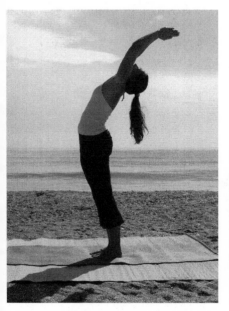

POSITION 11

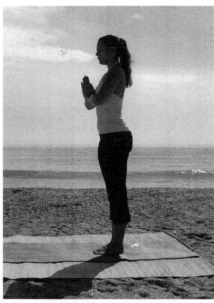

POSITION 12

straight. Your body should form a straight line, from head to toe.

6. Exhale and lower the knees to the floor. Keeping your abdomen and hips elevated, lower your chest to the floor, followed by your forehead. This position is known as *Sastanga Namaskar* or eight curved prostration; only eight portions of the body come in contact with the floor: two feet, two knees, two hands, chest, and forehead. Even the nose is kept off the floor if possible. Beginners may put the chin on the floor (instead of their foreheads) if necessary.

7. Inhale, lower the hips to the floor and bend back, arching the spine as much as possible. Bend your arms into your body and relax your shoulders.

8. Exhale, lifting the body to form an inverted "V". Your hands and feet should be flat on the floor and in the same place as the previous posture. Keep your elbows straight.

9. Inhale and bring your right foot between and level with your hands. Lower your left knee to the ground and arch up, lifting the chin and looking up.

10. Exhale and bring the left leg in line with your hands and right leg. The knees should be straight. Bring your head down to your knees as you did before.

11. Inhale and straighten up, stretching your arms over your head in one smooth motion. Bend backward as far as you can.

12. Exhale as you straighten up, bringing the palms back together at the heart chakra. Take a quick second to center yourself, then drop your arms and relax.

Initially, hold each pose as long as it takes you to feel firm and steady, and gradually decrease the amount of time you spend in each each pose. Optimally you should "flow" through the exercises in rhythm with your breath.

Liber Resh vel Helios

0. These are the adorations to be performed by aspirants to the A∴A∴.

1. Let him greet the Sun at dawn, facing East, giving the sign of his grade. And let him say in a loud voice:

Hail unto Thee who art Ra in Thy rising, even unto Thee who art Ra in Thy strength, who travellest over the Heavens in Thy bark at the Uprising of the Sun.

Tahuti standeth in His splendour at the prow, and Ra-Hoor abideth at the helm.

Hail unto Thee from the Abodes of Night!

2. Also at Noon, let him greet the Sun, facing South, giving the sign of his grade. And let him say in a loud voice:

Hail unto Thee who art Ahathoor in Thy triumphing, even unto Thee who art Ahathoor in Thy beauty, who travellest over the heavens in thy bark at the Mid-course of the Sun.

Tahuti standeth in His splendour at the prow, and Ra-Hoor abideth at the helm.

Hail unto Thee from the Abodes of Morning!

3. Also, at Sunset, let him greet the Sun, facing West, giving the sign of his grade. And let him say in a loud voice:

Hail unto Thee who art Tum in Thy setting, even unto Thee who art Tum in Thy joy, who travellest over the Heavens in Thy bark at the Down-going of the Sun.

Tahuti standeth in His splendour at the prow, and Ra-Hoor abideth at the helm.

Hail unto Thee from the Abodes of Day!

4. Lastly, at Midnight, let him greet the Sun, facing North, giving the sign of his grade, and let him say in a loud voice:

Hail unto Thee who art Khephra in Thy hiding, even unto Thee who art Khephra in Thy silence, who travellest over the heavens in Thy bark at the Midnight Hour of the Sun.

Tahuti standeth in His splendour at the prow, and Ra-Hoor abideth at the helm.

Hail unto Thee from the Abodes of Evening.

5. And after each of these invocations thou shalt give the sign of silence, and afterward thou shalt perform the adoration that is taught thee by thy Superior. And then do thou compose Thyself to holy meditation.

6. Also it is better if in these adorations thou assume the God-form of Whom thou adorest, as if thou didst unite with Him in the adoration of That which is beyond Him.

7. Thus shalt thou ever be mindful of the Great Work which thou hast undertaken to perform, and thus shalt thou be strengthened to pursue it unto the attainment of the Stone of the Wise, the Summum Bonum, True Wisdom and Perfect Happiness.[29]

Yoga Glossary

agni: One of the five tattwas—the element of fire.

aham: Ego.

Ahimsa: One of the tenets of Ashtanga Yoga's Yama; it means nonviolence or noninjury.

ajapa: Mantra repeated silently.

Ajna chakra: One of the seven major chakras; it's located in the area of the pineal gland behind the forehead. Also known as the psychic center.

akasha: The fifth element; ether or astral.

Anahata chakra: One of the seven major chakras; it's located in the area of the heart.

ananda: Bliss; ecstasy.

antar: Inner, internal.

antar kumbhaka: The part of the Pranayama cycle in which the breath is retained after inhalation.

Aparigraha: One of the tenets of Ashtanga Yoga's Yama; it means noncovetousness.

apas: One of the five tattwas—the element of water.

Ardha Padmasana: Half Lotus pose.

Asana: A Yoga position designed to facilitate the flow of energy in the body and mind. The practice of Asana also refers to the third part of Ashtanga Yoga which is concerned with the ability to sit in a comfortable, easy, firm upright position during meditation. The third limb of Ashtanga Yoga.

ashram: A place where people live together to practice Yoga. Most people stay in ashrams for a short amount of time, using them primarily to deepen their practice and their understanding of yogic philosophy.

Ashtanga Yoga: The eight-fold path of Yoga as outlined by Patanjali. See also Raja Yoga.

Asteya: One of the tenets of Ashtanga Yoga's Yama; it means nonstealing.

atman: Soul.

Aum: The sound that represents the outer, inner, and super conscious states.

bahir: Outside, external.

bahir kumbhaka: The part of Pranayama cycle in which the breath is held after exhalation.

bandha: Creating an energy lock in a specific area by contracting various muscles.

Bhagavad-Gita: A part of the famous Hindu epic "Mahabharata," in which Lord Krishna instructs his disciple Arjuna, explaining the concepts of Karma Yoga, Sannyasa Yoga, Jnana Yoga and Bhakti Yoga.

bhakti: Devotion.

Bhakti Yoga: The yogic practice of devotion.

Bhastrika Pranayama: A technique in which the breath is vigorously drawn in and out through the nose in equal proportions. Also known as "bellows' breathing."

Bhujangasana: Cobra pose.

Brahmacharya: One of the tenets of Ashtanga Yoga's Yama; it means "flowing with Brahma."

Brahman: Supreme consciousness; absolute reality.

chakra: An energy center in the body. There are seven major chakras located at various junctions within the nadis, or energy channels.

chandra: Moon.

chidakasha: Psychic space in front of the closed eyes, just behind the forehead.

chin mudra: Hand gesture in which the first finger is placed at the bottom of the thumb, the last three fingers are unfolded. It affirms awareness of the psychic state.

chit: Knowledge of self; consciousness.

Dhanurasana: Bow pose.

Dharana: The sixth limb of Ashtanga Yoga. The practice of concentration.

Dharma: Duty; righteous path.

Dhyana: The seventh limb of Ashtanga Yoga. Contemplation of the true nature of the subject the Yogi is focusing on.

diksha: Initiation conferred by a spiritual teacher or guru.

guna: Quality or nature. See also sattva, rajas, and tamas.

guru: Enlightened teacher or evolved soul who endeavors to enlighten and train his or her disciples.

Hatha Yoga: Branch of Yoga that is concerned with physical postures (asanas) or exercises.

Ida nadi: One of the three primary energy channels in the body. Ida runs along the left side of the spine from the Muladhara chakra to the Ajna chakra.

Isvarapranidhana: One of the tenets of Ashtanga Yoga's Niyama; surrendering one's destiny to a Higher Power.

japa: Vocalized repetition of mantra; chanting.

jnana: Knowledge; understanding; wisdom.

jnana mudra: Gesture in which the index finger is bent so that its tip is joined with the tip of the thumb, and the other three fingers are spread out.

Jnana Yoga: The Yoga of knowledge, attained through spontaneous self-analysis and investigation of abstract and speculative ideas.

kala: Light.

kapal: Cerebrum; skull.

Kapalabhati Pranayama: A breathing technique emphasizing rapid, forceful exhalations. Its practice clears the nasal passages of excess mucus and enlivens and sensitizes the spinal column.

karma: Effect; destiny or action; the act of doing.

Karma Yoga: The Yoga of action. Aims at supreme consciousness through action; discussed in Bhagavad-Gita.

Koormasana: Tortoise pose; an advanced posture.

kriya: Activity; an energetic yogic practice.

Kriya Yoga: The practice of Kundalini Yoga.

kumbhaka: Breath retention.

Kundalini: The life force.

Kundalini shakti: The primordial energy that lies curled like a serpent in the Muladhara chakra.

loka: World; universe; plane.

Makarasana: Crocodile pose.

Manipura chakra: One of the seven major chakras; it's located in the area behind the navel, at the solar plexus.

mala: A string of beads used to aid concentration during Mantra Yoga.

mantra: A form of sound; specifically a sacred word or phrase of spiritual significance and power.

Mayurasana: Peacock pose; an advanced pose that stimulates the Manipura chakra while strengthening the arms and improving general strength, balance, and concentration.

moksha: Liberation from the karmic wheel of birth and death.

Muladhara chakra: One of the seven major chakras; it's located in the area of the perineal floor. The lowest energy center in the human body where Kundalini originates.

mouna: Silence, especially the practice of silence.

mudra: A specific gesture used in meditation to place a psychic "seal" on the energies manipulated during practice.

nada: Sound.

nadi: Energy channels in the body, similar to the meridians in acupuncture.

niyama: Observance; discipline.

Om: See Aum.

Padmasana: Lotus pose; a seated meditative posture.

Param: Highest, supreme God.

Paramatma: God; the supreme atma.

Patanjali: Author of *The Yoga Sutras* and preacher of the eight-fold (Ashtanga) Yoga.

Pingala nadi: One of the three primary energy channels in the body. Pingala runs along the right side of the spine extending from the Muladhara chakra to the Ajna chakra.

prakamya: Fulfillment of desire.

prakasha: Inner light.

prakriti: Nature.

prana: A type of subtle energy that animates every living thing.

Pranayama: A technique of controlling the body's energy flow through breathing exercises.

prasad: An offering, either to or from the teacher or higher power.

Pratyhara: "Gathering toward oneself"; withdrawal of the senses from stimuli. The first stage of focusing the mind inward during meditation.

pravritti: Attached action; the path of active involvement in the world.

prithvi: One of the five tattwas—the element of earth.

puja: Ceremonial worship; ritual.

purnima: The day of the full moon.

purusa: Spirit; individual soul; pure consciousness of man.

Raja Yoga: Also known as Ashtanga Yoga. Yogic philosophy consisting of eight parts, or limbs: Yama, Niyama, Asana, Pranayama, Pratyhara, Dharana, Dhyana, and Samadhi.

rajas: One of the three gunas; its qualities are activity, energy, and passion.

rechaka: Exhalation.

Rudra: Shiva.

Sahasrara chakra: One of the seven major chakras; it's located at the crown of the head.

Samadhi: A state in which the practitioner becomes one with the object of meditation; supreme union with spiritual supraconsciousness. The last stage of Ashtanga Yoga.

Samtosa: One of the tenets of Ashtanga Yoga's Niyama; contentment, both with oneself and one's surroundings and circumstances.

sannyasa: A monk; one who has renounced the world to seek self-realization.

Sarasvati: "She of the stream"; the goddess of wisdom and consort of Brahma, presiding over the arts, speech, and knowledge.

Sarvangasana: Shoulder stand.

sastra: Scripture; treatise.

Sat: Existence; reality; life.

satguru: A guru who has attained self-realization.

sattva: One of the three gunas; its qualities are pureness, joy, and pleasure.

Satya: One of the tenets of Ashtanga Yoga's Yama; it means honesty or truth.

Sauca: One of the tenets of Ashtanga Yoga's Niyama; the cultivation of internal and external cleanliness.

shakti: Vital force; energy.

Shashankasana: Moon pose.

shisya: Disciple; student.

siddhi: Metaphysical powers obtained through Yoga practices.

Siddhasana: A meditative seated posture also called the Adept's pose or the "pose of perfection."

Sirshasana: An inverted pose. The body is balanced on the crown of the head.

Soma chakra: Minor chakra situated above Ajna chakra, contained within the Sahasrara chakra.

Sukhasana: Known as the "easy" pose or Cross-legged pose.

Surya nadi: See Pingala nadi.

Sushumna nadi: The major energy channel in the body. Sushumna is located in the center of the spinal cord.

Svadhisthana chakra: One of the seven major chakras; it's located in the area of the pelvis.

Svadhyaya: One of the tenets of Ashtanga Yoga's Niyama; self-awareness, introspection.

Tadasana: A standing posture known as the Tree pose.

tamas: One of the three gunas. Its qualities are inertia, laziness, and sluggishness.

Tapas: One of the tenets of Ashtanga Yoga's Niyama. It means self-discipline; paying attention to the needs of the body.

Upanisad: "To sit close by devotedly"; the last part of the Vedas, whose central teaching is that the nature of man is equal to that of Brahman, or the Absolute. According to the Upanisad, the entire purpose of life is the realization of Brahman.

Vajrasana: The Thunderbolt pose; commonly used in meditation. A kneeling posture with buttocks resting upon the heels.

Vajrayana: Another name for Tibetan Buddhism; the "diamond vehicle."

Vamacara: The left-hand way in Tantra.

vasita: Ability to subdue all objects to one's will.

vayu: One of the five tattwas—the element of air.

Veda: Knowledge; wisdom; inspired scripture. In Indian philosophy, there are four ancient texts—Rig, Yajur, Sama, and Atharva, which explain and regulate every aspect of life from supreme reality to worldly affairs. The Vedic texts are among the oldest books in the world.

Vishuddha chakra: One of the seven major chakras. It is located behind the base of the throat.

Yama: Abstention; control; restraint. Yama is the first limb of Raja Yoga. It's tenets are nonviolence, truth, nonstealing, moderation, and noncovetousness.

yantra: A geometrical diagram with mystical properties. Yantras can be used for meditation, worship, or protection.

Yoga: "Union"; yoke. A holistic spiritual path that leads to union with the Divine.

Yogacara: Practice of Yoga.

Yogin: "Joined or connected with"; one who practices Yoga.

Yogini: A female Yoga practitioner. Also, a witch, fairy, or sorceress.

Yoga nidra: "Yogic sleep"; a relaxed state in which the body and mind are deeply relaxed while possessing complete awareness.

yoni: Source; womb.

yuga: Aeon; time cycle.

NOTES

[1] Aleister Crowley, "Notes for an Astral Atlas" in *Magick: Liber ABA, Book Four* (Boston: Weiser Books, 1998), pp. 499–512.

[2] Vivekananda, *Raja Yoga: Introduction to Patanjali's Aphorisms* (New York: Ramakrishna-Vivekananda Center, 1970), p. 96.

[3] Swami Vishnudevanda, *The Complete Illustrated Book of Yoga* (New York: Bell Publishing Company, 1960), p. 51.

[4] Dion Fortune, *The Training and Work of an Initiate* (Boston: Weiser Books, 2000), pp. 109–110.

[5] Aleister Crowley, *Magick: Liber ABA, Book Four* (Boston: Weiser Books, 1998), p. 197.

[6] Fortune, *The Training and Work of an Initiate* (Boston: Weiser Books, 2000), p. 110.

[7] Ayurveda is a traditional, holistic East Indian healing modality.

[8] A yantra is a sacred geometrical lineal representation of a cosmic principle.

[9] The Svayambhu Lingam and the coiled serpent represent the potential energy of Shiva and Shakti.

[10] Bija mantras are the sacred Sanskrit letters assigned to each chakra and shown at the center of each yantra.

[11] In the Western symbol set the element of fire is represented by an upward pointing triangle, the flames rising (like the aspirations) toward the sky. The fluidity and interconnected nature of these symbols is instructive.

[12] The terms "heavens" and "earth" in this instance encompass more than their actual physical realms, extending to the multi-layered psychic planes as well.

[13] Harish Johari, *Chakras: Energy Centers of Transformation* (Rochester, VT: Destiny Books, 1986).

[14] Swami Kripalu, quote found online: *http://www.kripalu.org/pdfs/kyta_quotes.pdf.*

[15] *Vyasa Sutras*, Chapter IV, Section I, Verse 7

[16] Aleister Crowley, *Liber E vel Exercitiorum* is included in *Magick: Liber ABA, Book Four* (Boston: Weiser Books, 1998), pp. 604–612.

[17] The Lesser Banishing Ritual of the Pentagram in Liber O vel Manus et Sagittae, included in *Magick: Liber ABA, Book Four* (Boston: Weiser Books, 1998) pp. 613–626.

[18] Swami Vishnudevananda, *The Complete Illustrated Book of Yoga* (New York: Bell Publishing Company, 1960), p. 228.

[19] The Mudra of Harpocrates is given by pressing the right forefinger against the lips. This gesture is also known as the Sign of Silence.

[20] Dion Fortune, *Practical Occultism in Daily Life* (Wellingborough, Northamptonshire: Society of the Inner Light, 1981), p. 17.

[21] Aleister Crowley, *Magick: Liber ABA, Book Four* (Boston: Weiser Books, 1998), p. 20.

[22] Vivekananda, *Raja Yoga: Introduction to Patanjali's Aphorisms* (New York: Ramakrishna-Vivekananda Center, 1970), p. 72.

[23] Aleister Crowley, Liber III vel Jugorum is included in *Magick: Liber ABA, Book Four* (Boston: Weiser Books, 1998), pp. 647-650.

[24] Rumi, Jalal Al-Din, *Open Secret: Versions of Rumi,* translated by Coleman Barks (Boston: Shambhala Books, 1999) p. 7.

[25] Emerson, Ralph Waldo, *The Conduct of Life,* "Power." (Whitefish, MT: Kessinger Publishing, 2004).

[26] Aleister Crowley, These instruction on Dharana are taken from Liber E vel Exercitiorum, included in *Magick: Liber ABA, Book Four* (Boston: Weiser Books, 1998), pp. 604–612.

[27] Aleister Crowley, *Magick: Liber ABA, Book Four* (Boston: Weiser Books, 1998), p. 41.

[28] Rumi, Jalal Al-Din, *The Illustrated Rumi,* translated by Coleman Barks (New York: Broadway Books, 1997) p. 98.

[29] Aleister Crowley, Liber Resh vel Helios is included in *Magick: Liber ABA, Book Four,* (Boston: Weiser Books, 1998), pp. 655–656

BIBLIOGRAPHY

Austin, Miriam. *Yoga for Wimps*. New York: Sterling Publishing Company, Inc., 2000.

Avalon, Arthur, trans. *The Serpent Power*. Madras, India: Ganesh & Co. Private Ltd., 1964.

———. trans. *Tantra of the Great Liberation*. New York: Dover Publications, 1972.

Cavendish, Richard, ed. *Man, Myth & Magic*, Vol. 22. New York: BPC Publishing Ltd., 1970.

Crowley, Aleister. *Eight Lectures on Yoga*. Laguna Hills, CA: Thelema Media LLC, 1991.

———. *Magick: Liber ABA, Book Four*. Boston: Weiser Books, 1998.

Edgerton, Franklin, trans. *The Bhagavad-Gita*. New York: Harper & Row, 1964.

Epstein, Gerald M.D. *Healing into Immortality: A New Spiritual Medicine of Healing Stories and Imagery*. New York: Bantam Books, 1994.

———. *Healing Visualizations: Creating Health Through Imagery*. New York: Bantam Books, 1989.

Fortune, Dion. *Practical Occultism in Daily Life*. Wellingborough, Northamptonshire: Society of the Inner Light, 1981.

———. *The Training and Work of an Initiate*. Boston: Weiser Books, 2000.

Grimes, John. *A Concise Dictionary of Indian Philosophy*. Albany, NY: State University of New York Press, 1996.

Hawksley, L. & I. Whitelaw, eds. *101 Essential Tips: Yoga*. London: Dorling Kindersley, 1995.

Johari, Harish. *Chakras: Energy Centers of Transformation*. Rochester, VT: Destiny Books, 1986.

———. *Tools for Tantra*. Rochester, VT: Destiny Books, 1988.

Johnston, Charles, trans. *The Yoga Sutras of Patanjali*. London: John M. Watkin, 1964.

Leadbeater, Charles.W. *The Chakras*. Wheaton, IL: Quest Books, 1985.

Le Mée, J., trans. *Hymns from the Rig-Veda*. New York: Alfred A. Knopf, 1975.

Müller, F. Max, trans. *The Upanisads*. New York: Dover Books, 1962.

Regardie, Israel. *Foundations of Practical Magic*. Wellingborough, Northamptonshire: The Aquarian Press Ltd., 1983.

———. *Healing Energy, Prayer, and Relaxation*. Las Vegas: Golden Dawn Publications, 1989.

Rivière, J. Marquès. *Tantrik Yoga*. New York: Samuel Weiser Inc., 1970.

Vishnudevananda, Swami. *The Complete Illustrated Book of Yoga*. New York: Bell Publishing Company, 1960.

Vivekananda, S. *Raja Yoga*. New York: Ramakrishna-Vivekananda Center, 1970.

Wasserman, James. *Aleister Crowley and the Practice of the Magical Diary*. Boston: Weiser Books, 2006.

———. *The Mystery Traditions: Secret Symbols and Sacred Art*. Rochester, VT: Destiny Books, 2005.

To Our Readers

Weiser Books, an imprint of Red Wheel/Weiser, publishes books across the entire spectrum of occult and esoteric subjects. Our mission is to publish quality books that will make a difference in people's lives without advocating any one particular path or field of study. We value the integrity, originality, and depth of knowledge of our authors.

Our readers are our most important resource, and we appreciate your input, suggestions, and ideas about what you would like to see published. Please feel free to contact us, to request our latest book catalog, or to be added to our mailing list.

Red Wheel/Weiser, llc
500 Third Street, Suite 230
San Francisco, CA 94107
www.redwheelweiser.com